Perioperative Care for Organ Transplant Recipient

Edited by Alexander Vitin

Published in London, United Kingdom

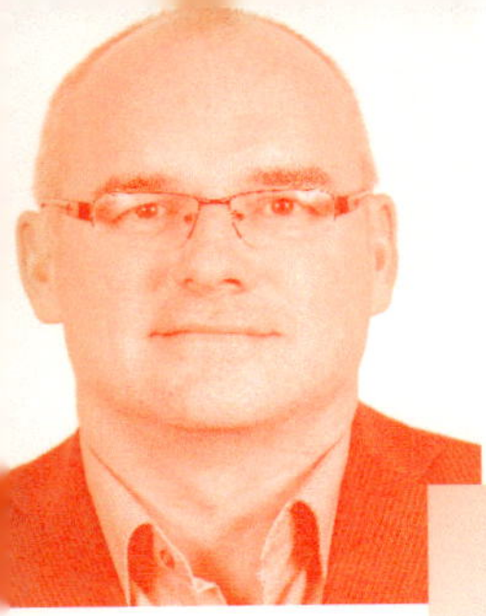
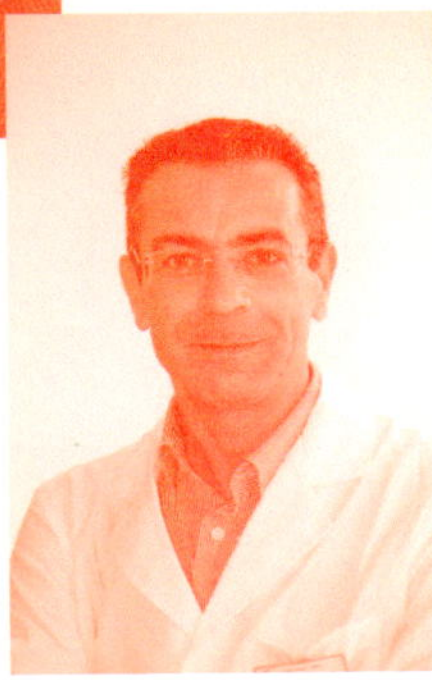
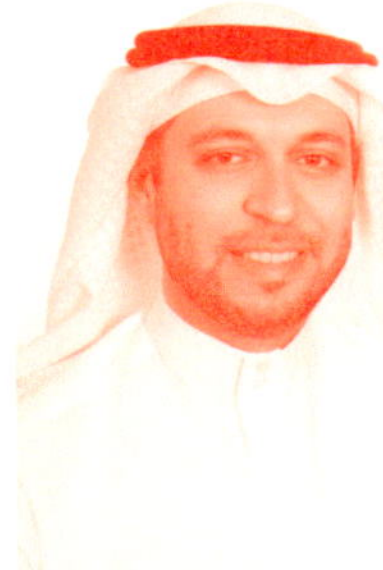
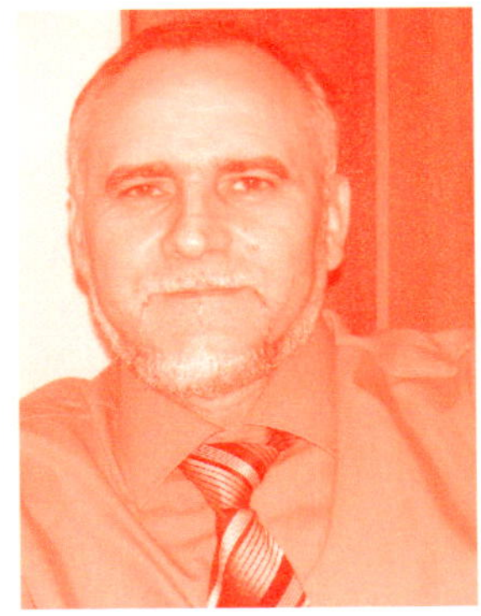
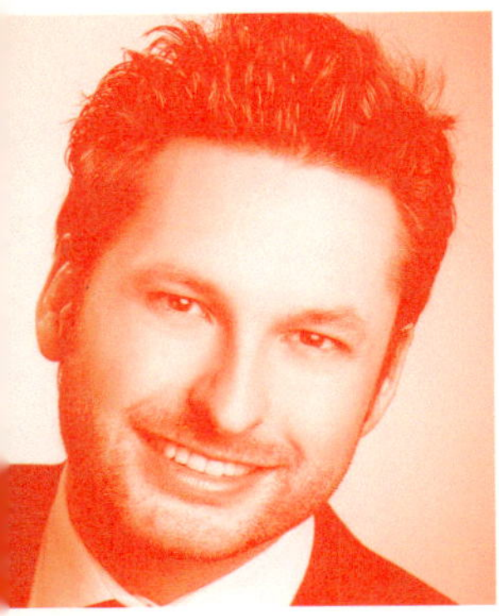
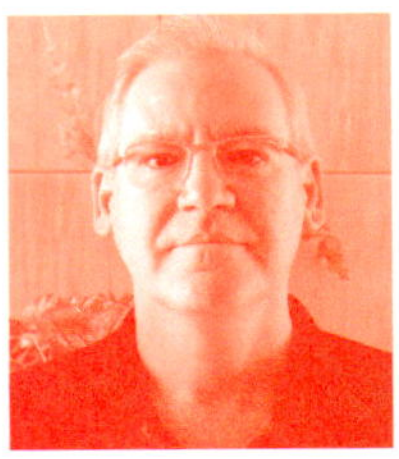
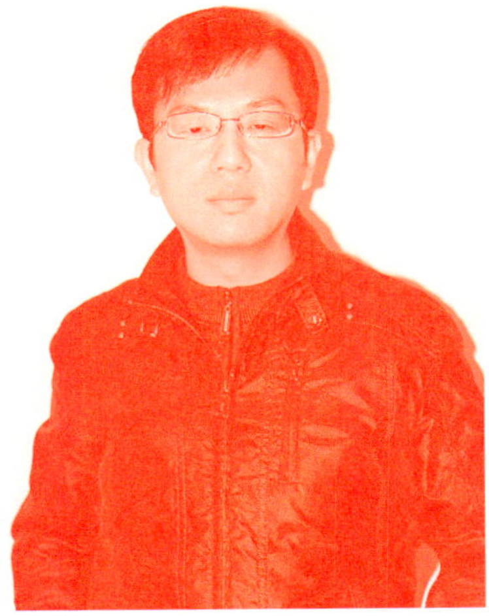

IntechOpen

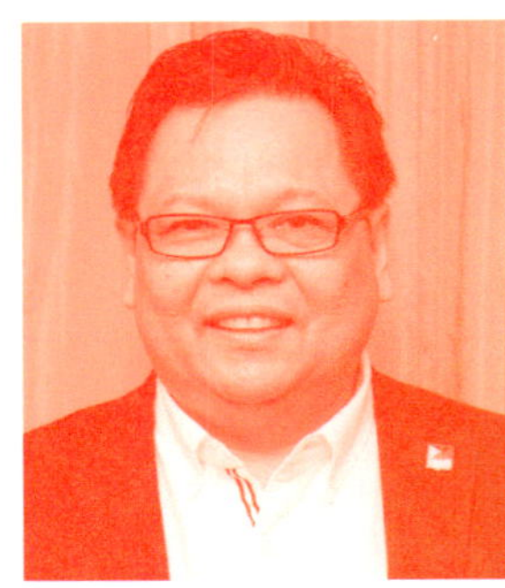
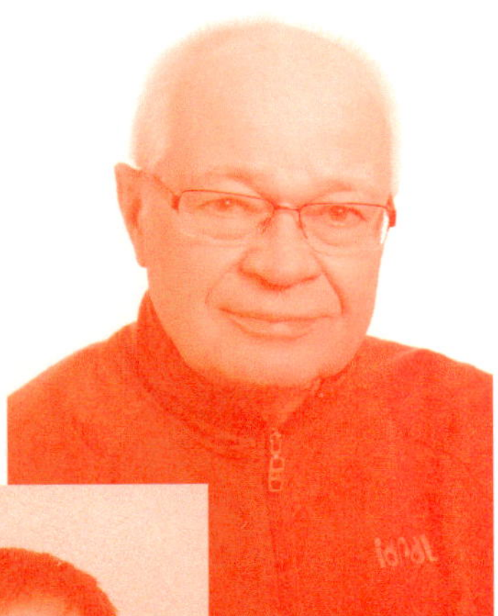
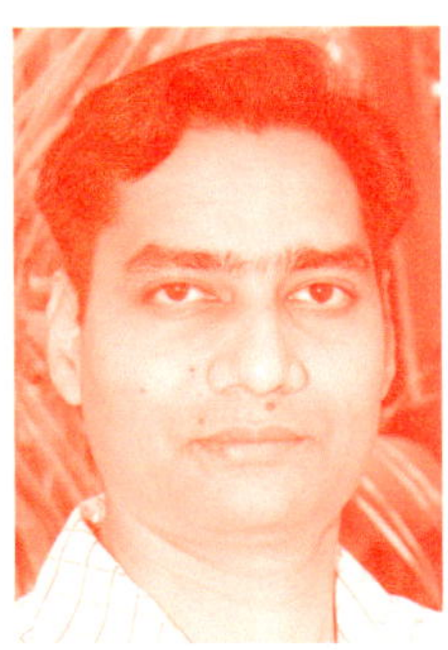
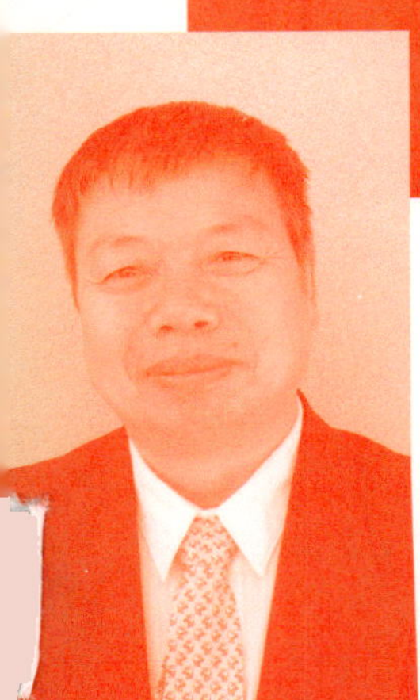
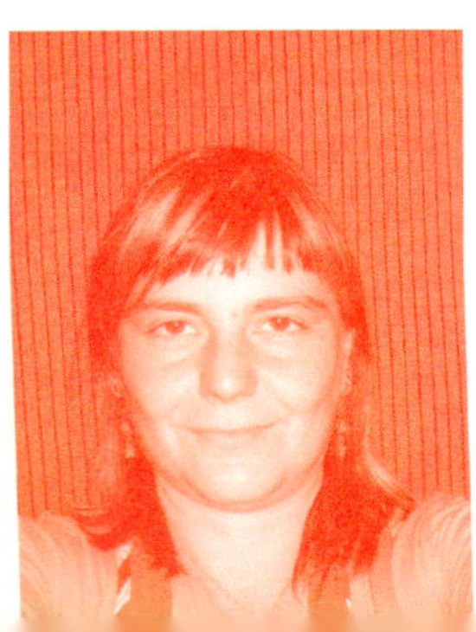
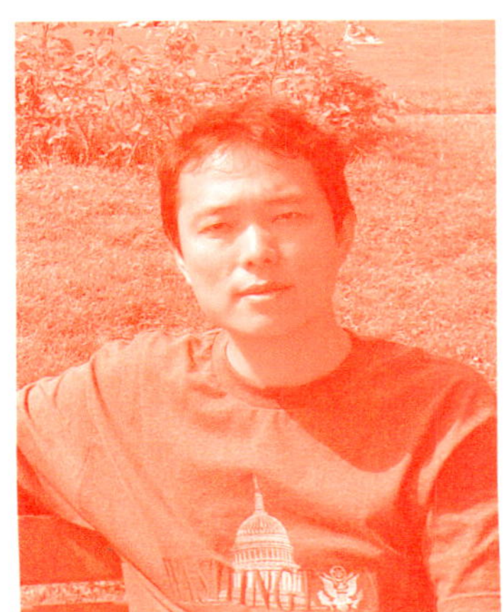

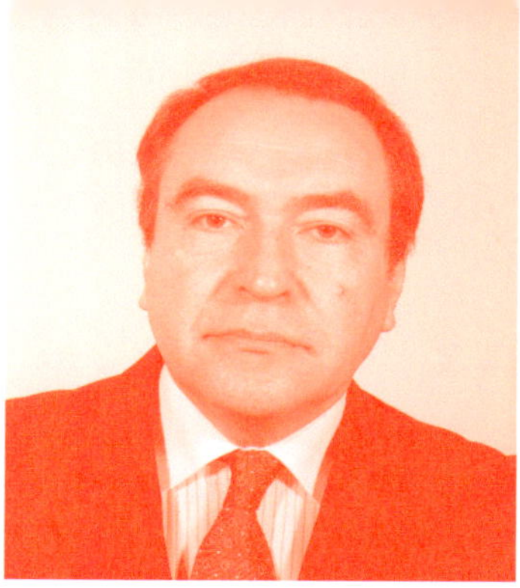
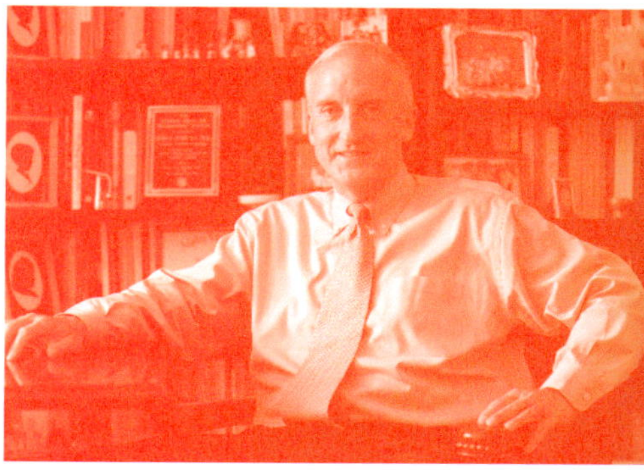
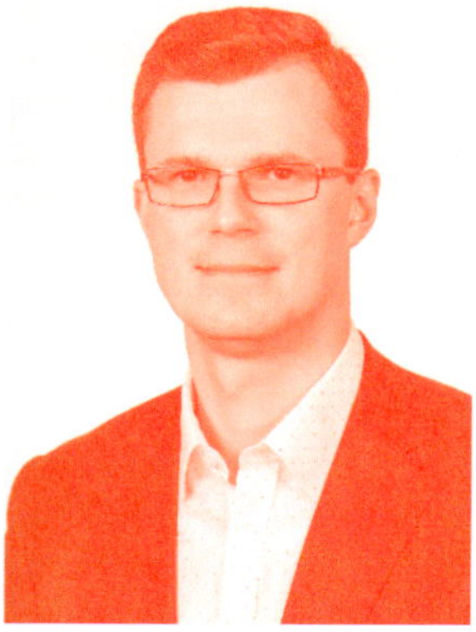
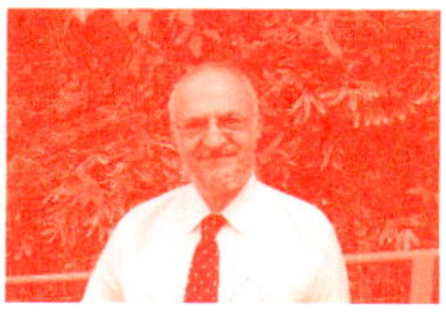
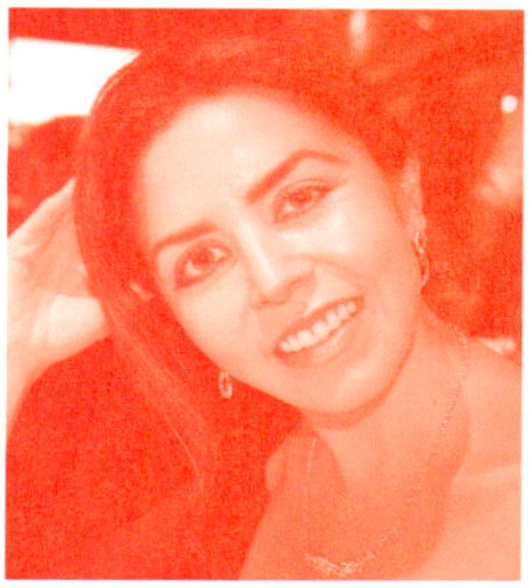

Supporting open minds since 2005

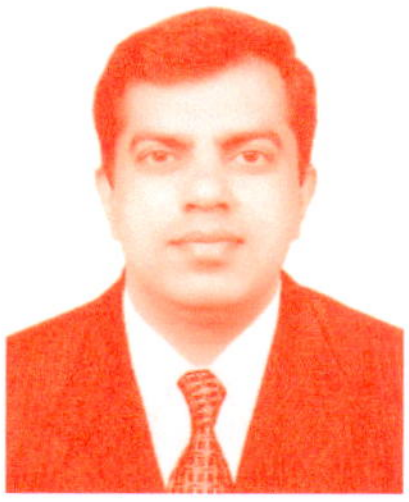
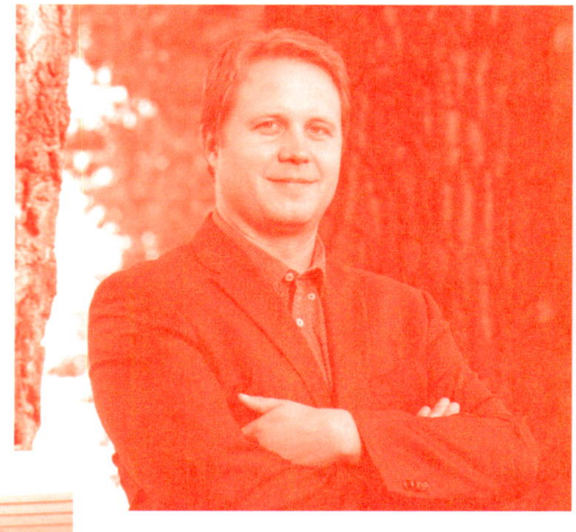
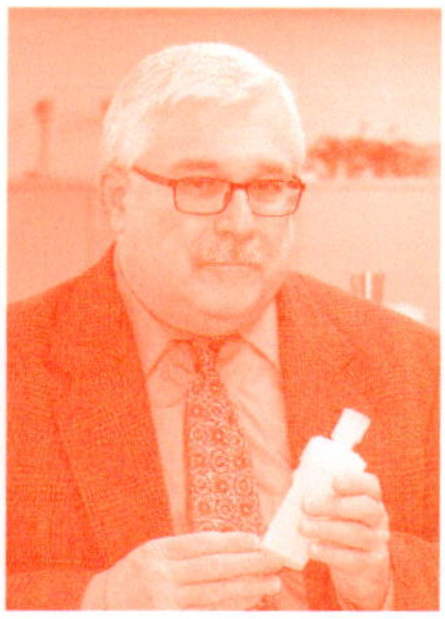
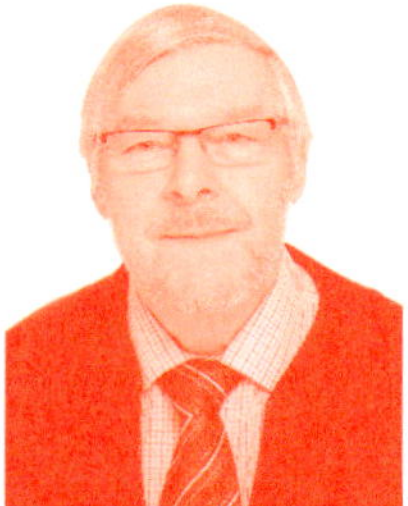
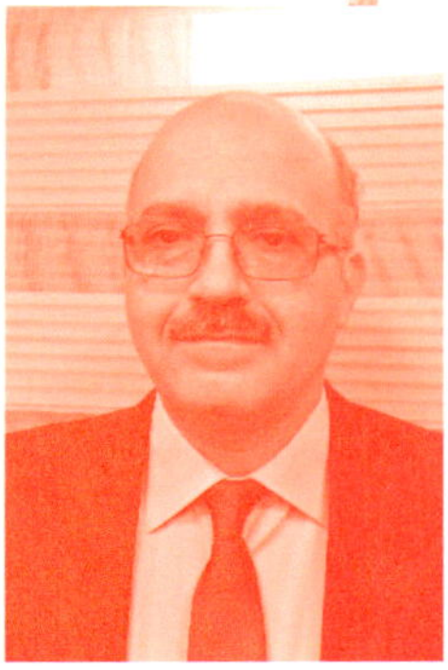
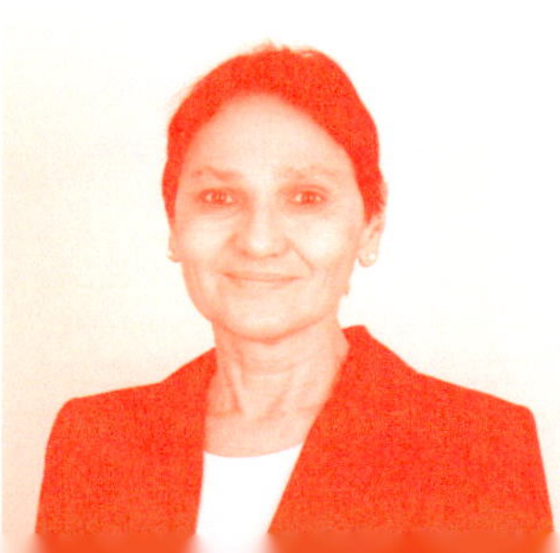
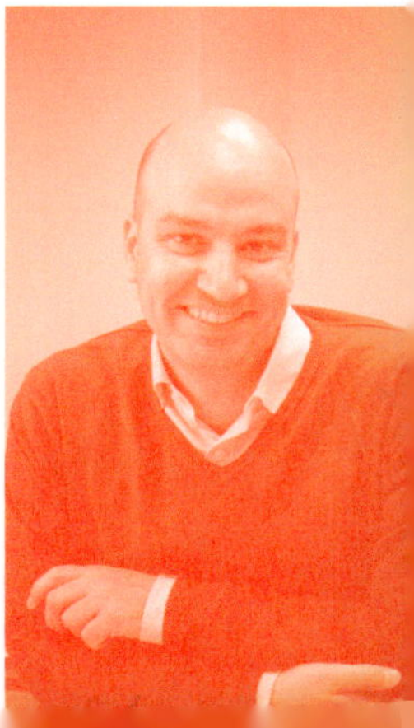

Perioperative Care for Organ Transplant Recipient
http://dx.doi.org/10.5772/intechopen.77696
Edited by Alexander Vitin

Contributors
Stacey Brann, Steven Geier, Olga Timofeeva, Ross Francis, David Johnson, Carmel Hawley, Sebastian Hultin, Wickii Vigneswaran, John Hallsten, Željka Večerić-Haler, Nika Kojc, Clark Kensinger, Jon S. Odorico, Alexander Vitin

First published in London, United Kingdom, 2019 by IntechOpen
IntechOpen is the global imprint of INTECHOPEN LIMITED, registered in England and Wales, registration number: 11086078, The Shard, 25th floor, 32 London Bridge Street
London, SE19SG – United Kingdom
Printed in Croatia

British Library Cataloguing-in-Publication Data
A catalogue record for this book is available from the British Library

Additional hard and PDF copies can be obtained from orders@intechopen.com

Perioperative Care for Organ Transplant Recipient
Edited by Alexander Vitin
p. cm.
Print ISBN 978-1-78984-422-1
Online ISBN 978-1-78984-423-8
eBook (PDF) ISBN 978-1-83962-242-7

For EU product safety concerns:
IN TECH d.o.o., Prolaz Marije Krucifikse Kozulić 3, 51000 Rijeka, Croatia, info@intechopen.com or visit our website at intechopen.com.

Meet the editor

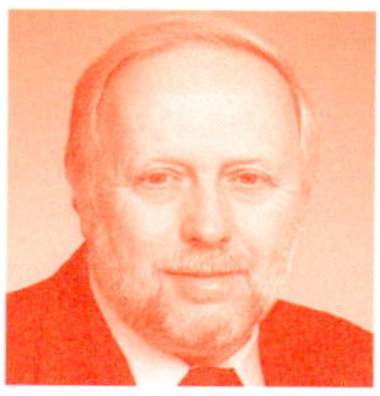

Dr. A. Vitin, MD, PhD, graduated cum laude from Kharkiv Medical University in 1981. He completed his PhD on the topic of Extracorporeal Detoxication Procedures in End-Stage Liver Disease Patients in 1986. He started to work as an ICU and as an attending anesthesiologist in 1987. From 2003, he worked as a faculty (now at the rank of associate professor) and attending anesthesiologist in the Department of Anesthesiology and Pain Medicine, University of Washington, Seattle, WA, USA. He is the author of more than 40 publications in peer-reviewed journals, several books, and book chapters. He has presented the results of his research work at scientific congresses in seven countries. Anesthesia and perioperative care for organ transplant recipients are his main areas of expertise and scientific interest.

Contents

Preface

Ever since the very first successful solid organ transplants, transplantation-related science has displayed exponential growth. Physicians and researchers from many specialties are becoming more involved in transplantation medicine, which has exceeded the boundaries of one medical specialty and become a whole new field of medical science. There are more than 75 periodic issues, among which are more than 40 high-impact journals, publishing the results of research work from all over the world. A PubMed search alone returns about 800,000 titles of indexed publications pertinent to the field of transplantation, which covers approximately 70% of the total published work worldwide. There are also numerous books, book chapters, and other publications on the field of transplantation-related topics that find their readers every year. Ongoing research is funded by tens of millions of dollars and euros; these funds come from government and private investors, and are surpassed probably only by cancer and heart research funding.

And yet, among countless publications covering most of the areas in this particular field, specific segments such as perioperative care for the organ recipient remain underrepresented, and many topics are still not covered. The resulting lack of large, prospective studies, along with the relative scarcity of conceptual-level review articles, has prompted the choice of the main topic of this book, with intention to fill in the gap by collecting and presenting articles dedicated to these ignored problems.

This book is addressed to physicians and researchers working in the ever-expanding research and practice fields of transplantation medicine.

Its purpose is to present the transplantation community with a collection of works written by prominent experts in a variety of transplant-related fields, encompassing the most recent scientific and practical developments and accomplishments in the highly specialized segment of transplantation medicine, such as perioperative care for organ transplant candidates and recipients.

Alexander A. Vitin, MD, PhD
Associate Professor,
Department of Anesthesiology and Pain Medicine,
University of Washington,
Seattle, WA, USA

Director,
Transplant Anesthesia,
UW Medical Center,
USA

Section 1

Introduction

Chapter 1

Introductory Chapter: Tour De Force of Transplantation Science

Alexander A. Vitin

1. Overview

As one of the relatively young, yet already well-established medical disciplines, transplantation medicine encompasses a wide variety of clinical subspecialties. The concept of failing organ replacement with the donor's or an artificial one has found its way into literally every clinical field, where one or multiple organ insufficiency and eventual failure are concerned. Ever-increasing number of the patients on the waiting lists, rapidly growing demand for donor organs, already well-proved efficiency of organ transplantation as an ultimate treatment for end-stage organs' failure, and ever-expanding infrastructure of transplantation industry are factors promoting the explosive growth of the transplantation industry. The foundation of this industry rests on two pillars: transplantation medicine and transplantation science, with substantial overlapping and blurred boundaries. The sheer immensity of transplantation industry may be best illustrated by very impressive statistics and facts, accomplishments, and ongoing research trends [1–5].

At present, organ and tissue transplantation procedures of any kind are being performed in more than 111 countries, which cover about 81% of world population, and new countries are joining this club every year. Close to 140,000 organs are being transplanted every year worldwide. According to most recently published OPTN data (May 22, 2019), in the USA alone during the period of 31 years (from January 11, 1988 to April 30, 2019), close to half million (451,847, to be precise) kidney, 166,383 liver, 73,216 heart, 38,989 lung, 23,959 kidney-pancreas, and numerous other organ transplantations have been performed in more than 80 transplant programs, and the exponential increase of these numbers constitutes the current trend.

Fifteen international and more than 140 local/countrywide organizations in more than 111 countries are incessantly doing a great job in coordinating efforts in the areas of research promotion, development, and improvement of practical aspects of organ donation and transplantation process. Dozens of scientific meetings in many countries worldwide provide stage for scientists and physicians to present results of research, share experience, and exchange opinions.

Ever since the very first successful solid organ transplants (1954, first successful kidney transplant; 1967, first successful liver and heart transplants), transplantation science remains in the state of rapid exponential growth. Physicians and researchers from literally every imaginable specialty are getting more and more involved in transplantation medicine, which long ago overgrew the boundaries of one particular medical specialty and became a whole new field of medical science. Results of clinical and experimental research provide a plenty of material for myriad publications worldwide every year. There are easily more than 75 periodic issues, among which are more than 40 high-impact journals, publishing results of countless research works from all over the world. PubMed search alone returns about 800,000 titles of the indexed publications, pertinent to the field of transplantation, which covers approximately 70% of the total published works on the transplantation-related topics worldwide. There are also numerous books, book chapters, and other publications on these topics, that find their readers every year. Ongoing research is funded by tens of millions dollars and euros; these funds are coming from various government organizations and private investors, surpassed probably only by cancer and heart research funding.

And yet, among countless publications, covering most areas in this particular field, such a specific segment of key importance as perioperative care for the organ recipient remains underrepresented, and many topics of it still uncovered. The resulting lack of big, prospective studies, along with relative scarcity of conceptual level review articles, has prompted us to choose the main topic of this book, with the true intention to fill in the gap by collecting and presenting the articles dedicated to at least some of the under-covered problems.

2. Components of perioperative care

Perioperative care for organ transplant candidate/recipient is an exceedingly complex and multifaceted enterprise. It comprises three main components.

A. Preoperative care begins from selection of the proper candidate. In today's realm of organ transplantation, the current trend of performing combined, more complicated organ transplants on ever-increasing number of sick patients with severe cardiopulmonary, renal, endocrine co-morbidities, once considered as posing insurmountably high risk, prohibitive for surgery, is quickly becoming an everyday reality. At this stage, a person's medical and surgical history and current disease status, treatment progress, success or lack thereof, and compliance with numerous medication regimes are being reviewed. The critical portion of the selection includes a great deal of current functional status assessment, ability to tolerate multiple challenges of organ transplant surgery and postoperative period, and, most importantly, prediction of outcome, immediate and long-term. There are numerous prediction algorithms and systems, such as MELD score for liver transplant candidates, for example. The degree of functional impairment (after all, majority of patients suffer from end-stage organ failure, sometimes severe multi-organ insufficiency) is a matter of continuous re-assessment and optimization, whenever appropriate and feasible, in preparation to actual organ transplantation surgery. Numerous diagnostic studies, some of which invasive, are employed at this stage to pinpoint the problem and track the treatment progress.

This stage also includes an assessment of patient's mental status, habits, lifestyle, social and financial aspects, geographical factors, housing and transportation particulars, availability of family support in the posttransplant period, coping skills and intellectual capacity, illicit drug use and alcohol consumption, and many other pieces of the information, necessary to make an initial selection, and keep the candidacy active.

The organ transplant surgery is a culmination of the transplantation process, the central and most important part of the whole enterprise. The very possibility of the surgery is contingent on availability, oftentimes immediate, and proper quality of the donor organ. Current policies and practices of organ donation and sharing, procurement and conservation techniques comprise a huge field of scientific and practical knowledge, and their discussion is beyond the scope of this book.

B. Intraoperative care for organ transplant recipient, even in the relatively straightforward cases, is by far one of the most challenging tasks the anesthesiologist ever encounters in his/her practice. The spectrum of problems and challenges include choice of particular anesthesia technique (that depends on organ failure involved and other patient-related factors), significant, sometimes life-threatening hemodynamic disturbances and acid-base/electrolytes disbalance, major ongoing blood loss, massive blood products administration, coagulation deficit correction, necessity of temporary organ replacement techniques (such as intraoperative dialysis), use of case- and organ-specific technologies and modalities, such as use of vasoactive agents for hemodynamic optimization, TEE, ECMO, total circulatory arrest, and plenty more. Some of the most challenging aspects of anesthesia care for transplant recipient include unpredictability of the timing (it is literally 24/7, no exclusions) and length of procedures, and, with ever-growing body of practical experience, incidence of unanticipated, rare complications, such as stress cardiomyopathy or intraoperative myocardial infarction. For all these reasons, and more, transplant anesthesiology has been established as one of the major independent subspecialties in the field of anesthesiology.

Immediate postoperative care is an inseparable part of this stage. The challenges here, albeit quite similar to those encountered in the operating room, are different in many ways (time resolution, for one). The reasons of major morbidity and mortality of freshly transplanted patient include variety of cardiovascular complications; primary transplanted organ dis- and non-function; super-acute rejection; and numerous surgery-specific complications, such as hemorrhage, vascular thrombosis, dehiscence, bronchial anastomosis leaks, biliary leaks, wound infections/septic state, and also plenty of seemingly trivial, matter-of-everyday-practice problems, such as hemodynamic instability, blood glucose fluctuations, acid-base disturbances, ventilator-associated problems, pulmonary complications (pulmonary edema, ARDS, pneumonias, atelectasis), and early cognitive dysfunctions—all of which require immediate and apt attention and incessant efforts directed on correction, as soon and as complete as possible.

C. Later, posttransplant care encompasses the time period from recipient's discharge form critical care unit until discharge from the hospital. The time frame for this stage varies (the range is from days to months), due to transplanted organ-, surgery-, related specifics, early complications and other medical conditions. At this stage, clinicians face quite different and very specific set of challenges, which includes choice and maintenance of immunosuppressive therapy; early, late, sub-acute, and chronic rejections; late organ dysfunctions; transition from pretransplant organ-specific hemodynamic profile to normalized one; wide variety of infectious complications (opportunistic bacterial, viral, and fungal infections); exacerbations of chronic diseases; early malignancies; PTSD and other mental, mood, and memory problems, and more. Albeit already not as acute and severe as major immediate perioperative problems, these conditions nevertheless remain as important and, oftentimes, as deadly, and certainly bear an enormous weight on the short- and long-term patient and organ survival and well-being.

Deep understanding and detailed knowledge of these components, their mutual influences, connections, and interactions are necessary conditions for any further progress in this particular field, both in scientific and practical aspects.

3. The book's concept and purpose

The presented book is addressed to physicians and researchers, working in the ever-expanding research and practice fields of transplantation medicine.

This book's purpose is to present the transplantation community with the collection of works performed and articles written by prominent experts in the variety of transplant-related fields, encompassing most recent scientific and practical developments and accomplishments in the highly specialized segment of transplantation medicine, such as perioperative care for organ transplant candidate and recipient.

While considering the inclusion of broad, well-researched, albeit constantly discussed, topics, such as candidacy/selection criteria, indications for transplant, hemodynamic management, coagulopathy, renal failure, diabetes in transplant recipient and more, as undoubtedly beneficial, it should be stressed though, that the very intent of this book is rather to focus on problems and issues, encountered while providing intra-(anesthesia) and postoperative critical care for patients, undergoing single and combined organ transplant surgery.

Considering and actually making a perioperative care specifically for organ transplant recipient a conceptual base for the selection of scientific, research- and practical-oriented articles is not an easy task. The amount of mutually influencing factors; interactions; and seemingly far-fetched, but, after close examination, very relevant pieces make such a selection work quite arduous, taking into account the sheer volume of already published excellent works in the field of transplantation science. It is our hope, however, that the collection of outstanding articles, containing most updated, pertinent, and highly relevant information, presented in this book, will help explore new horizons of knowledge, inspire new ideas for research projects, and promote practical improvements and developments.

Author details

Alexander A. Vitin
Department of Anesthesiology and Pain Medicine, University of Washington Medical Center, Seattle, WA, USA

*Address all correspondence to: vitin@uw.edu

References

[1] Mar C, Álvarez M, Marco J, Mahíllo B, Gil D, et al. Global Organ Transplant Activities in 2015. Data from the Global Observatory on Donation and Transplantation (GODT). Abstracts, S29. Transplantation: August 2017. DOI: 10.1097/01.tp.0000525015.43613.75

[2] Transplants By Organ Type January 1, 1988 - April 30, 2019 Based on OPTN data as of May 22, 2019. Available from: https://optn.transplant.hrsa.gov/data/view-data-reports

[3] Data repots WHO Global Observatory on Donation and Transplantation (GODT). Available from: www.transplant-observatory.org

[4] Organ Donation and Transplantation. Available from: https://ec.europa.eu/health/blood_tissues_organs/events/journalist_workshops_organ_en

[5] Mahillo B, Carmona M, Álvarez M, Noel L, Matesanz R. Global database on donation and transplantation: Goals, methods and critical issues. Transplantation Reviews (Orlando). 2013;**27**(2):57-60. DOI: 10.1016/j.trre.2013.01.001. Epub 2013 Mar 9. Available from: www.transplant-observatory.org

Section 2

Kidney Transplant: Problems and Solutions

Chapter 2

Perioperative Care for Kidney Transplant Recipients

Sebastian Hultin, Carmel M. Hawley, David W. Johnson and Ross S. Francis

Abstract

Transplantation carries significant mortality benefit compared to dialysis in end-stage kidney disease. Increased perioperative risk, however, results in a higher mortality in the first 3 months post-transplantation compared to remaining on haemodialysis. Consequently, optimal perioperative management is essential. Patients presenting for kidney transplantation require rapid assessment and preparation for theatre to minimise ischaemic times and improve mortality and graft outcomes. This task is often complicated by the presence of multiple medical comorbidities. Furthermore, early complications of hypotension, delayed graft function, renovascular and ureteric surgical complications and rejection render the perioperative phase of transplant challenging for the recipient and for the transplant team. In this chapter, we outline current practices in the assessment and management of kidney transplant recipients during the perioperative period, particularly focusing on their clinical application and the evidence underpinning them.

Keywords: comorbidity, kidney transplantation, perioperative care, risk assessment, treatment outcome

1. Introduction

Non-communicable diseases now account for 75% of deaths globally, with chronic kidney disease (CKD) rapidly rising up the ranks as a cause of death, reaching eleventh on the list in 2016 [1]. The estimated global crude prevalence of CKD in 2016 was 275.9 million cases associated with a crude mortality of 1.2 million [2].

As CKD patients' renal function declines, mortality rises to an estimated lifespan of 8 years for patients on dialysis of 40–44 years of age and 4.5 years to patients 60–64 years of age. Improvements in dialysis therapy have been accompanied by a decline in mortality rate [3]. Despite this, the long-term mortality on dialysis remains significantly inferior to that following kidney transplantation.

A systematic review in 2011 identified 110 studies including nearly 2 million patients with transplantation conferring a mortality advantage over dialysis. Only studies with follow-up periods <3 months favoured dialysis, attributed largely to perioperative complications and higher immunosuppression post-transplantation [4]. Accordingly, transplant and dialysis registry studies have confirmed increased mortality in transplanted patients compared to dialysis at 3 months (HR 2.0, 1.5–2.7, $p < 0.001$) with reversal at 6 months (HR 0.27, 0.16–0.47, $p < 0.001$) with 80% reduction in mortality following transplantation compared to dialysis at 12 months [5].

The increase in mortality associated with kidney transplantation highlights the need for optimal perioperative management to minimise the risks and maximise the benefits associated with transplantation. This chapter focuses on the principles and evidence of perioperative management of transplant patients.

2. Pre-operative transplant management

2.1 Initial clinical assessment pre-transplant

Patients on the kidney transplant waiting list have usually undergone a thorough medical and surgical assessment prior to listing to identify significant comorbidities that would preclude transplantation. Optimisation of cardiovascular comorbidities, including diabetes mellitus (DM) and hypertension, is important not only for prevention of cardiovascular disease but also for avoidance of hypertensive and diabetic damage to the transplanted graft. Nevertheless, at the point that an intended recipient is admitted to hospital for transplantation, a thorough reassessment is important to identify any new medical issues, as well as to ensure that the recipient is sufficiently medically stable for a general anaesthetic and surgery.

On arrival at the transplanting hospital, bloods are collected with a request for the laboratory to process these urgently (**Table 1**). In addition, a chest radiograph and ECG are performed.

While these investigations are being processed, a medical history and examination should be undertaken with the patient with the aim of documenting:

- Any new medical comorbidities, in particular symptoms suggesting the development of vascular disease (angina, claudication, peripheral ulceration), malignancy (unexpected weight loss, new mass or lymphadenopathy) or active infection (fever, constitutional symptoms).

- Signs or symptoms of fluid overload, with assessment of the patient's weight in relation to their recent clinic weights (or current target weight if on dialysis).

- The patient's usual daily urine volume.

The presence of potential new medical comorbidities should prompt review of suitability for, and safety of proceeding with transplantation. The development of ischaemic heart disease, vascular disease, malignancy or active infection would preclude proceeding with transplantation.

Blood tests:
Renal and liver chemistry including phosphate, calcium, and LDH
Full blood count
Coagulation profile
Blood group + hold
Serum for tissue typing investigations
Serology for CMV, EBV, VZV, toxoplasma hepatitis B, hepatitis C, HIV
Pregnancy test as appropriate
Urine culture unless anuric
Chest radiograph
Electrocardiogram

Table 1.
Usual investigations for a patient presenting for kidney transplant.

A key decision during the assessment is whether a patient requires dialysis prior to transplantation. Similarly, donor factors associated with a high probability of delayed graft function (e.g., donation after circulatory death [DCD] kidney, prolonged anticipated cold ischaemic time) require a lower threshold for dialysis. Significant hyperkalaemia (a typical threshold may be a serum potassium concentration > 5.5 mmol/L) or fluid overload should prompt urgent dialysis prior to transplantation. In general, it is better to control fluid and electrolyte abnormalities effectively with dialysis pre-operatively rather than to attempt dialysis in a less stable patient post-surgery. Due to tissue damage and intraoperative bleeding, hyperkalaemia may worsen post-operatively. If haemodialysis is required prior to transplantation, patients are usually slightly above their target weight with the aim of avoiding intraoperative hypotension. Minimal or no heparin should be administered during dialysis to minimise the risk of perioperative haemorrhage.

2.2 Management of pre-existing medication

Patients with advanced kidney disease are often on multiple medications, many of which can be safely discontinued at the time of transplantation, including most antihypertensive medication, phosphate binders, cinacalcet, and erythropoiesis-stimulating agents. However, some medications should usually be continued as follows:

- Active vitamin D compounds in patients post-parathyroidectomy are usually continued. Calcium levels post-transplant follow a biphasic pattern with early decline in the post-operative week without supplementation. The protective effect of raised PTH is absent in patients post-parathyroidectomy, thereby risking precipitating severe hypocalcaemia if such patients are not supplemented with active vitamin D compounds (calcitriol and alfacalcidol) [6].

- Beta blockers are usually not stopped abruptly in the perioperative period due to concerns that this may lead to rebound tachycardia and increase the risk of mortality [7]. However, it may be reasonable to reduce the dose and/or convert patients to a beta blocker with a shorter duration of action (e.g., metoprolol) to reduce the risk of hypotension in the post-operative period.

- Statins, although generally safe, can predispose to rhabdomyolysis if used in conjunction with CYP450-3A4 inhibitors [8]. We suggest ceasing statins until outside the perioperative period.

- Antiplatelet therapy with aspirin is usually continued perioperatively, and many transplant centres routinely prescribe aspirin to recipients who are not already receiving this agent to reduce the risk of transplant vessel thrombosis, although this has a poor evidence base [9]. Dual antiplatelet therapy with aspirin plus agents, such as platelet P2Y12 receptor inhibitors (e.g., clopidogrel and ticagrelor), would usually be considered a contraindication to transplantation, both because of the increased risk of bleeding and the frequent association of significant vascular disease in patients requiring this combination.

- Erythropoiesis stimulating agents (ESA) may be continued on the basis of some studies identifying anaemia as an independent predictor of mortality in the intermediate post-transplant period [10]. There are, however, no studies showing benefits of continued ESA therapy or defining optimal haemoglobin targets [11]. European Best Practices Guidelines for anaemia management recommend that ESA not be ceased in patients undergoing surgery, but no specific recommendations are made regarding transplantation [12].

Potential transplant recipients who are anti-coagulated with warfarin require urgent reversal of anticoagulation prior to surgery. There are often local protocols for warfarin reversal, but a typical approach would be 1–2 mg oral vitamin K administered as soon as the patient presents to hospital, followed by infusion of either fresh frozen plasma or a prothrombin complex concentrate, such as prothrombinex-VF, depending on the INR [13]. Whether intravenous heparin is required post-operatively will depend on the strength of the indication for anti-coagulation, the degree of post-operative haemorrhage, and a decision regarding this should be made in consultation with the transplant surgeons. Where the risk of thrombosis is not excessively high, it is preferable to defer recommencing warfarin until at least 4 weeks post-transplant due to the frequent requirement for a transplant biopsy during this period.

Although non-vitamin K oral anticoagulants (NOACs) are currently not used routinely in end-stage kidney disease (ESKD) patients, indications for their use have been expanding into patients with more severe renal dysfunction. Nonetheless, NOACs should be avoided in ESKD patients on the active transplant list.

2.3 Pre-operative management of diabetes and hyperglycaemia

In Australia, over 23% of patients who are listed for a deceased donor transplant have diabetes [ANZDATA 2016]. The presence of autonomic neuropathy should be noted, as this may help predict haemodynamic instability and risk for graft hypoperfusion post-operatively. Similarly, gastroparesis may have important implications for immunosuppressive drug absorption if severe and retinopathy may complicate post-operative medication management if visual acuity is substantially reduced.

After admission for kidney transplantation, patients with type 2 diabetes should omit hypoglycaemic medication during the period of preoperative fasting, with regular capillary glucose monitoring performed every 1–2 h. Hypoglycaemia is managed with intravenous dextrose. If significant hyperglycaemia develops, an intravenous insulin infusion is the safest method to control glucose levels until the recipient is able to eat post-operatively. Patients with type 1 diabetes should commence an intravenous insulin infusion after admission to hospital to prevent the development of ketoacidosis.

2.4 Immunosuppression

After the decision has been made to proceed with a transplant, an immunosuppression regimen is selected. This regimen is usually initiated before the recipient goes to theatre so that immune function is attenuated prior to donor antigen exposure after reperfusion of the allograft. The choice of immunosuppressive regimen is individualised depending on the circumstances of the recipient and, in particular, the perception of immunological risk (**Table 2**).

Most patients undergoing kidney transplantation will receive induction immunosuppression, typically consisting of intravenous methylprednisolone combined with either a monoclonal antibody targeting CD25 (the high affinity α-chain of the IL-2 receptor) [14], such as basiliximab, or a lymphocyte-depleting antibody (such as thymoglobulin [15] or alemtuzumab [16–18]). Induction therapy is combined with ongoing maintenance immunosuppressive therapy, typically consisting of

Very low risk	Identical twin donor
Low risk	HLA-identical sibling donor, no DSA
Average risk	HLA-mismatched donor, no DSA
High risk	HLA-mismatched donor, detectable DSA, negative cross-match or ABO-incompatible donor following desensitisation
Very high risk	HLA-mismatched donor, detectable DSA, positive cross-match

DSA, donor-specific antibody.

Table 2.
Immunological risk assessment for kidney transplantation.

three immunosuppressive agents [19]. The most commonly prescribed combination in Australia and the USA currently is tacrolimus, mycophenolate and prednisolone [20, 21]. ABO-incompatible transplants as well transplants where there is a pre-transplant DSA requiring plasma-exchange prior to transplantation are outside the scope of this chapter. Similarly, special circumstances including steroid-free immunosuppression are not discussed here.

2.5 Prophylactic medications

The administration of immunosuppression needs to be balanced against the increased risk of infection. With ESKD patients being routinely subjected to hospital environments, additional consideration should be given for prophylaxis in patients colonised with multi-resistant organisms. Patients with prior known serious or recurrent infections should be evaluated carefully and assessed for recurrence and presence of occult infection prior to proceeding with transplantation. In addition, gastro-protection, infection and VTE prophylaxis is charted (**Table 3**).

Despite some controversy for the use of surgical antibiotic prophylaxis, routine prescribing is common, generally following local practices and guidelines [22]. No consensus currently exists for optimal antibacterial prophylaxis, but the general approach is to minimise dose and duration of administration to prevent emergence of antibiotic resistance [23]. A Cochrane systematic review is currently being undertaken to evaluate the evidence for antibiotic prophylaxis in preventing postsurgical site infections in solid organ transplant recipients [24]. Where there are risk factors that may predispose the recipient to bacterial transmission from the donor, such as treated bacteraemia or urine infection, the duration of antibiotic prophylaxis is adapted to cover the appropriate organisms.

Prior to introduction of prophylaxis, PJP was an important cause of severe pneumonia, associated with an estimated 29–50% mortality [25]. Since the widespread use of co-trimoxazole prophylaxis, the incidence of PJP has declined to an estimated incidence of 0.8 case per 1000 person at 1-year post-transplant [26]. Co-trimoxazole prophylaxis is routinely prescribed in most transplant centres for 6–12 months post-transplant and many centres now advocate for continued prophylaxis following PJP outbreaks [27]. If co-trimoxazole is contraindicated, alternative agents are inhaled pentamidine isethionate or oral dapsone.

Prophylaxis against urinary tract infections (UTIs) is usually provided by the co-trimoxazole therapy administered for PJP prophylaxis. On the basis of limited evidence, perioperative UTI prophylaxis is recommended and in the case of co-trimoxazole intolerance, another agent could be chosen [11].

Systemic anti-fungal prophylaxis is not routinely administered to kidney transplant recipients [28]. However, oral nystatin or amphotericin is frequently

Gastro-protection	Ranitidine (or PPI) therapy while on high dose steroids
Bacterial prophylaxis	Perioperative antibiotic therapy prescribed based on local guidelines and adapted for recipient multi-resistant organism colonization or potential donor infection
PJP prophylaxis	6–12 months co-trimoxazole. Consider lifelong therapy
UTI prophylaxis	6 months co-trimoxazole
Oropharyngeal candidiasis prophylaxis	Oral nystatin or amphotericin for duration of admission. Optimal duration uncertain
Systemic fungal prophylaxis	Not generally prescribed due to low incidence of invasive fungal infection
CMV prophylaxis	Oral valganciclovir. Duration depending on donor and recipient serostatus—see **Table 4**
VTE prophylaxis	Unfractionated heparin and mechanical calf compressors unless contraindicated until patient mobile

Table 3.
Perioperative prophylaxis.

prescribed in the early post-operative period to reduce the risk of oropharyngeal candida infection [11]. The optimal duration of therapy is unknown, largely due to low event rates, but a typical approach would be therapy for the first month post-transplant [29].

Previous cytomegalovirus (CMV) infection is common, with a seroprevalence of up to 75% in transplant recipients [30]. The risk of developing CMV viraemia post-transplant depends on the serostatus of both donor and recipient as well as the induction immunosuppression agent (**Table 4**). The highest risk CMV infection is seen in seronegative recipients of a transplant from a seropositive donor, and is increased in patients treated with T cell depleting agents [31].

Several antiviral agents have been shown to reduce the risk of CMV infection (with the added benefit of also providing prophylaxis against herpes simplex and herpes zoster reactivation) in transplant recipients, including intravenous ganciclovir and oral acyclovir and valganciclovir, irrespective of donor status and induction immunosuppressive regimen [32]. Unfortunately, viral prophylaxis has shown little benefit in reducing the incidence of EBV-related PTLD [33]. Sustained prophylaxis benefit is observed with longer duration therapy (>3 months) with the main adverse effects being leukopenia with longer therapy duration [32]. Due to the observed benefit in reducing the incidence of CMV disease and cost effectiveness, 6 months antiviral prophylaxis is generally prescribed in high-risk CMV D+R− pairs [34]. An accepted alternative approach to universal prophylaxis is to monitor for CMV viraemia regularly post-transplant and initiate pre-emptive therapy should significant viraemia develop [32, 35].

Due to the gastro-erosive effects of prednisolone, ranitidine 150 mg twice daily for gastro-protection is usually recommended, noting the potential risk of interstitial nephritis and chronic kidney disease with proton-pump inhibitors (PPIs) [36, 37]. If ranitidine is contraindicated or ineffective, use of low dose PPIs as second line is recommended.

Deep venous thrombosis (DVT) has not been extensively evaluated in the literature. Kidney transplantation is categorised as a moderate risk group of patients for development of thromboprophylaxis conferring an estimated risk of DVT of 6% [38]. Limited studies have suggested the incidence to be lower with mechanical thromboprophylaxis alone [39]. Despite the lack of evidence, thromboprophylaxis

CMV D−R−	Usually no prophylaxis
CMV D+R+ or D−R+	Valganciclovir for 3 months
CMV D+R−	Valganciclovir for 6 months
D, donor serostatus; R, recipient serostatus.	

Table 4.
Prophylaxis for cytomegalovirus.

is generally initiated immediately post-operatively in the absence of contraindications or concerns of active haemorrhage. A combination of unfractionated heparin prophylaxis and mechanical calf compression is used, following local guidelines.

3. Intra-operative and immediate post-operative considerations

Although surgical and anaesthetic approaches and considerations are outside the scope of this chapter, intra-operative events have significant impacts on patient and graft outcomes. Review and documentation of intra-operative and immediate post-operative factors can help predict and guide subsequent clinical course (**Table 5**).

Any surgical complications or anatomical challenges (notably presence of multiple renal arteries, difficult bench surgery and renal capsule tear) should be communicated by the transplant surgeons as these can help predict perioperative complications. If available, intraoperative Doppler assessments should be documented to confirm adequate post-perfusion flow parameters in the transplanted kidney. Where there is perioperative concern regarding allograft perfusion, or early unexpected oligoanuria, an early duplex ultrasound may be requested to confirm flow in the transplant vessels.

Significant blood loss, requirement of inotropic support and intra-operative haemodynamic instability indicate suboptimal organ perfusion and are risk factors for delayed graft function (Section 5.4). Central venous line is placed at the time of surgery, and central venous pressure (CVP) is still used intra-operatively and in the immediate post-operative period. It is important to acknowledge controversies in absolute CVP targets, with studies advocating improved outcomes with high CVP (10–15 mmHg) targets at reperfusion [40, 41] and others observing increased kidney dysfunction with CVP >11 mmHg [42]. In general, intra-operative CVP trends can inform fluid management, but should not form the basis of a fluid management strategy due to inconsistent correlation with intravascular volumes [43].

Despite preoperative optimization, hyperkalaemia is common post-operatively due to tissue trauma and resorption of intra-abdominal blood. The presence of

Donor graft	Graft anatomy, backbench surgery, renal capsule tear
Graft perfusion	Appearance on cross-clamp release. Intraoperative Dopplers
Haemodynamics	Blood pressure profile, CVP, need for inotropic support, blood loss volume
Fluid balance	Volume of intravenous fluid administration during procedure, urine output
Biochemistry	Intraoperative insulin dextrose. Post-operative renal chemistry panel including urea, creatinine and potassium
Assessment of listed factors helps guide and predict perioperative management	

Table 5.
Post-operative documentation.

hyperkalaemia >6 mmol/L in the immediate post-operative period should prompt consideration of dialysis depending on the urine output. If graft urine output (with native residual renal function deducted) is >100 mL/h, it may be reasonable to manage the patient medically with insulin-dextrose infusion and loop diuretics. It should also be noted that intraoperative use of insulin-dextrose often results in rebound hyperkalaemia postoperatively.

4. Perioperative fluid management

Optimal fluid management strategy is contentious, although there is good evidence that fluid loading to maintain cardiac output and optimise renal perfusion, improves outcomes [44]. Intra-operative blood losses and fluid balance can be estimated through discussion with the transplant surgeon and anaesthetist and review of anaesthetic chart (Section 3). Currently, no studies on fluid management in the perioperative phase of renal transplantation exist to guide practice. A recent randomised trial demonstrated non-inferiority of a non-restrictive perioperative intravenous fluid strategy in high-risk abdominal surgery in terms of disability-free survival. Furthermore, the restrictive fluid strategy was associated with increased rates of acute kidney injury (8.6 vs. 5.0%. $p < 0.001$) [45]. Although generalizability to renal transplantation is uncertain, a restrictive fluid strategy should be avoided.

A common strategy for managing post-operative fluid replacement in the hours after kidney transplantation is to replace the urine output from the previous hour plus 30 mL to account for insensible losses. A loop diuretic and/or mannitol is sometimes administered during the transplant surgery to precipitate a diuresis, decreasing requirement for dialysis, but has not been shown to improve graft outcomes [46].

Frequent clinical assessment of the recipient's fluid status, including the jugular venous pressure, heart rate, blood pressure and urine output, is important to ensure adequate fluid replacement and to avoid volume overload. Traditional parameters and clinical assessment of fluid status, however, may be unreliable due to compromised homeostatic mechanisms in ESKD and the post-ischaemic transplanted kidney [47]. As soon as it is feasible post-transplant, recipients should be weighed with comparison to their preoperative weight as an objective guide to fluid status.

There is currently no evidence supporting one type of intravenous fluid therapy over another, although a pragmatic, registry-based, multi-centre, double-blind, randomised controlled trial comparing balanced crystalloid solution (PlasmaLyte) with 0.9% saline on the incidence of delayed graft function in 800 adults and children with end-stage kidney disease (ESKD) receiving a deceased donor kidney transplant in Australia and New Zealand is currently underway (ACTRN12617000358347).

A good urine output in the early post-transplant period is a helpful indicator of early graft function, although it may not be possible to differentiate allograft urine output from native urine output in recipients who have significant residual renal function. Oligoanuria may be an indicator of delayed graft function or a harbinger of an early complication, especially if the urine output was good initially (Section 5.4). An urgent ultrasound is a useful investigation to assess perfusion of the allograft at the bedside and to check for evidence of ureteric or vascular complications. The presence of hypoechoic fluid collections may indicate haemorrhage or urinary anastomotic leak (Section 5).

Blood tests to monitor serum creatinine and electrolytes are collected immediately post-transplant and then 6–12 h to monitor renal function and exclude hyperkalaemia. Some recipients may develop a significant diuresis, passing over a litre of urine per hour, and in this situation, frequent monitoring of blood tests 4–6 h is recommended to avoid over or under replacement of electrolytes.

5. Early complications

Complications in the perioperative phase are diverse, reflecting pre-existing transplant recipient comorbidities as well as individual surgical challenges. With the potential for there to be few symptoms from the denervated graft, most centres follow a protocol of investigations for early identification of post-transplant complications (**Table 6**).

Generally, an early renal transplant duplex ultrasound can identify vascular or anastomotic complications including renal vessel thrombosis or compression. The resistive index (RI) (measured peak systolic velocity—end diastolic velocity/ peak systolic velocity), normally, between 0.60 and 0.80, with levels >0.8 suggesting abnormal perfusion of the allograft, is a widely reported measure of allograft perfusion for duplex scans but does not seem to correlate well with renal histology [48]. A positive correlation has been reported between RI and recipient mortality, and the strongest predictor of an elevated RI was recipient age, suggesting that RI may be an indicator of recipient vascular disease [48]. Consequently, although the RI is commonly reported, clinicians need to be aware of its limitations.

Similarly, nuclear medicine imaging, such as a mercaptoacetyltriglycine (MAG3) or diethylenetriamine pentaacetic acid (DTPA) renogram, can assist in the assessment of allograft perfusion and early graft function as well as identify a ureteric anastomotic leak. Radionucleotide scanning may give an indication of the likely duration of delayed graft function [49, 50].

5.1 Haematological, biochemical and metabolic derangement

Electrolyte abnormalities are a frequent occurrence in the early post-transplant period. Perioperative hyperkalaemia is often followed by hypokalaemia due to diuretics and polyuria combined with large volume IV fluid replacement. Hypomagnesaemia is exacerbated by the tubular effects of CNI therapy and is associated with an increased risk of post-transplant diabetes [51, 52]. Hypophosphatemia is almost universal as a consequence of elevated FGF23 and PTH levels [53, 54]. To reduce the chance of arrhythmias, intravenous electrolyte replacement should target potassium levels in the normal range (3.5–5 mmol/L) and a serum magnesium >0.4 mmol/L. Hypophosphatemia is not usually associated with adverse clinical sequelae, but if severe (<0.4 mmol/L) can also be managed with intravenous replacement. Many transplant recipients require ongoing oral replacement of potassium, magnesium and occasionally phosphate in the first few weeks post-transplant, although this may be limited by gastrointestinal adverse effects.

Blood tests:
Twice daily full blood count and serum biochemistry
Alternate day CNI levels
Daily capillary glucose levels—if abnormal, manage as diabetes mellitus
Post-operative chest radiograph
Duplex ultrasound imaging, usually at days 2–4 post-transplant
MAG3/DTPA renogram as indicated by clinical progress

Table 6.
Common post-operative surveillance investigations.

Myelosuppression is commonly observed in post-transplant patients receiving immunosuppressive therapy. Myeloid, lymphoid and erythroid lineages can separately be affected in combination. Investigations focus on identification of the underlying cause for the haematological abnormality, and blood films are often helpful.

Post-operative anaemia is observed in around 40% of kidney transplant recipients due to erythropoietin deficiency, pre-transplant anaemia and intra-operative blood loss [55]. Initial management should focus ruling out haemorrhage as discussed in Section 5.2. The administration of an erythropoiesis-stimulating agent may be appropriate in recipients with poor initial graft function [11].

Lymphopenia and neutropenia are also common after transplantation, typically as a consequence of the medication-related bone marrow suppression associated with anti-proliferative agents (mycophenolate and azathioprine), mTOR inhibitors (sirolimus and everolimus) and antiviral agents such as valganciclovir for CMV prophylaxis [56–58]. G-CSF is typically administered if the absolute neutrophil count falls below 1000/μL (1.0×10^9/L) to try to avoid a severe neutropenia (neutrophil count <500/μL, or < 0.5×10^9/L), which is associated with a significant risk of severe infections and requires reverse barrier nursing [59]. Alternative causes of neutropenia should also be considered including parvovirus B12 and CMV infection [60].

Thrombocytopenia is comparatively less common, often occurring in conjunction with leukopenia due to bone marrow suppression as previously discussed. More severe thrombocytopenia is a risk factor for bleeding, and platelet transfusion may be necessary if invasive procedures, such as a renal biopsy, are required and the platelet count is <50×10^9/L [61]. An important consideration, if thrombocytopenia is observed post-transplant, is to look for any other evidence of thrombotic microangiopathy (TMA, **Table** 7) [62]. TMA occurring after transplant may be due to recurrence of primary haemolytic uraemic syndrome, or a de novo problem. Many triggers for de novo TMA post-transplant have been reported, including medication (CNI therapy, particularly in combination with mTOR inhibitors; valacyclovir), and infections (CMV, parvovirus B19) have all been associated with TMA with the potential for graft damage and kidney injury [63–65].

The post-operative stress response, combined with induction corticosteroid and cyclosporine or tacrolimus therapy, can result in significant perioperative hyperglycaemia even in patients who do not have pre-existing diabetes, with a reported incidence as high as 80–90% in some studies [67, 68] with post-transplant diabetes persisting in 10–45% depending on the definition used [69–73]. Hyperglycaemia is also associated with rejection in the perioperative period and in the long term carries adverse metabolic outcomes [74]. It is, therefore, important to monitor capillary glucose levels in all patients after kidney transplantation. Due to the contributions of immunosuppressive medications, and depending on other metabolic risk factors (pre-existing impaired glucose tolerance or diabetes, ethnicity, age and obesity)

- Thrombocytopenia—platelet count <150×10^9/L
- Microangiopathic haemolytic anaemia (MAHA)—haemoglobin <10 g/dL with evidence of red cell fragments on blood film (schistocytes)
- Elevated lactate dehydrogenase
- Elevated reticulocyte count
- Elevated bilirubin
- Reduced haptoglobin

Table 7.
Features of thrombotic microangiopathy on laboratory tests [66].

and immune risk, immunotherapy should be individualised [11]. A detailed discussion of the management of post-transplant hyperglycaemia and diabetes is beyond the scope of this chapter.

5.2 Hypotension: haemorrhage, sepsis and cardiac dysfunction

Perioperative hypotension is common and may reflect inadequate intravascular volume, vasoplegia induced by anaesthetic or analgaesic agents or cardiac dysfunction. Management involves perioperative fluid status optimization with judicious administration of fluid boluses while excluding alternative causes of hypotension including haemorrhage, sepsis and cardiac dysfunction. Recipients with persistent hypotension, despite what appears to be adequate fluid replacement, may require temporary inotropic support. Hypovolaemia, even in the absence of hypotension, increases the risk of delayed graft function resulting in worse graft outcomes [75, 76]. As coronary artery disease is common in patients with ESKD, ruling out ischaemic myocardial damage with ECG review and cardiac enzyme assay measurements is essential (Section 5.3).

Haemorrhage is common in the early period of kidney transplantation, frequently occurring within 48 h of surgery with a reported incidence of 15% [77]. Apart from hypotension, bleeding may manifest clinically with increasing surgical drain output, pain or swelling at the site of the transplant or a falling haemoglobin on serial blood tests. Risk factors for perioperative bleeding include difficult bench surgery, uraemic platelet dysfunction and administration of antiplatelet agents or heparin (either as thromboprophylaxis or during haemodialysis). In a retrospective analysis, difficult bench surgery was identified as the most significant risk factor for post-operative haemorrhage with a 4-fold increased risk. The use of antiplatelet drugs pre-transplant conferred a 2-fold increased risk. Additionally, dialysis vintage was also a risk factor, and each year on dialysis was associated with a 2% increased bleeding risk [77].

In the early post-operative phase, clinical features suggestive of haemorrhage should prompt urgent review of haematology profile, and consideration of imaging in liaison with the transplant surgeon. Peri-nephric hematomas may be identified on ultrasound, but deep or retroperitoneal haemorrhage may be difficult to identify requiring computed tomography. The development of a peri-nephric haematoma may lead to allograft compression, which if significant, may impair graft perfusion with increased diastolic pressures despite normal, or near normal, arcuate artery blood flow indices.

Management of perioperative bleeding requires administration of crystalloid fluids together with judicious transfusion of packed red cells to maintain adequate haemodynamic and haemoglobin targets. Transfusions should be minimised as much as possible, as perioperative blood transfusion leads to recipient sensitization and can increase the likelihood of de novo DSA formation [78]. The decision to proceed to surgical drainage should be individualised, following discussion with the transplant surgeon. The presence of a large haematoma, ongoing haemodynamic instability or features suggesting compression of the allograft, would usually lead to surgical re-exploration.

Sepsis should also be considered in the setting of unexplained hypotension. A high index of suspicion for infection should be maintained at all times since transplant recipients may not develop a fever, leukocytosis or raised inflammatory markers because of their immunosuppressed state (Section 5.7).

5.3 Cardiovascular complications

Due to the significant cardiovascular disease burden and risk associated with chronic kidney disease, cardiovascular complications post-renal transplantation are common. In a retrospective cohort study, the most common perioperative cardiovascular complication was arrhythmia (53%), followed by myocardial infarction (26.4%) with congestive heart failure being relatively rare (1%) [79, 80].

Hypertension, although often overlooked as a perioperative complication, is common, occurring in 50–70% of recipients. It is likely driven by multiple factors including pre-existing hypertension associated with ESKD, cessation of previous antihypertensive therapy at the time of transplantation, iatrogenic fluid administration to optimise allograft perfusion, calcineurin inhibitor therapy (CNI) and corticosteroid-related fluid retention [81]. Modification of fluid status, diuretic therapy and administration of dihydropyridine calcium channel blockers are common initial strategies used to control BP in the early post-transplant period. The non-dihydropyridine agents (diltiazem and verapamil) may be used, but have significant interactions with CNI (cyclosporine > tacrolimus) increasing CNI exposure. Angiotensin-converting enzyme inhibitors and angiotensin receptor blockers are usually avoided in the perioperative period to due to their potential to increase creatinine levels but can be introduced once allograft function has stabilised with appropriate monitoring of creatinine and potassium levels.

Despite pre-transplant screening for ischaemic heart disease, acute coronary syndromes (ACS) are still seen in the peri-transplant period, an indication of the limited sensitivity of non-invasive cardiac testing to detect clinically significant coronary disease in the ESKD population [82, 83]. ACS are a difficult complication to manage in the perioperative setting due to competing clinical priorities, and the potential benefits of antiplatelet and anticoagulant therapy need to be balanced against the risk of bleeding. Evaluation of the impact of the infarct on ventricular function can be assessed by echocardiography. Decisions on the optimal management including the potential need for angiography should be discussed with the local cardiology team.

Pre-existing congestive cardiac failure should be identified pre-transplantation and optimised through high-quality dialysis to control uraemia and volume overload as well as medical therapy. Large fluctuations in blood pressure and inter-dialytic weight gain will adversely affect myocardial function through cardiomyopathic remodelling and vasoactive humoral-mediated increases in vascular tone and damage. It is important to acknowledge controversies surrounding optimal blood pressure targets in dialysis patients and to individualise both blood pressure target and pharmacological hypertensive therapy [84, 85].

5.4 Delayed graft function

Delayed graft function (DGF) is a form of acute kidney injury and is usually defined as the need for dialysis post-transplant. DGF is associated with a higher incidence of acute rejection as well as poorer allograft survival, with a reported 40% greater risk of allograft loss and higher mean serum creatinine concentration [86, 87]. The reported frequency varies significantly (from 2 to 50%) due to heterogeneity of recipient and donor factors and definition of the event [75]. In Australia and New Zealand, nephrologist reported DGF is present in 19.5% of cadaveric renal transplants [ANZDATA 1997–2014].

Post-operative oliguria, failure of improvement of serum creatinine or the need for dialysis should prompt investigations to identify reversible causes of acute kidney injury, including assessment of risk factors for ATN, recipient hypotension or hypovolaemia, presence of post-surgical vascular or urological complications and rejection. In addition to a review of fluid status, haemodynamic parameters and the timing of a decrease in urine output, the following testing should be considered:

- Repeat serum biochemistry and haematology profile to rule out pre-renal kidney injury from anaemia and sepsis, taking account of haemoglobin and haematocrit fluctuations with fluid status dilution and unpredictable inflammatory response in the context of immunosuppression.

- Repeat CNI trough levels and review of CNI dosing and trends. These are nephrotoxic and may necessitate adjustment depending on the immune risk of the transplanted patient.

- Ultrasound duplex scan to rule out renovascular pathology. This also allows exclusion of peri-nephric collections and obstructive uropathy.

- Functional nuclear medical imaging, such as a MAG3, scan will allow assessment of perfusion, graft tracer uptake, and excretion.

- A renal biopsy is usually undertaken if DGF persists at day 5 post-transplant to rule out rejection, and is repeated weekly until there are signs of improving allograft function.

It is also helpful to consider risk factors associated with DGF in order to risk stratify and anticipate the clinical course of the transplanted patient (**Table 8**) [75].

In the setting of DGF, ongoing dialysis is often required. In haemodialysis patients, every effort should be made to preserve haemodialysis access. If haemodialysis is delivered through a central vascular catheter, this access should be preserved for this purpose alone and additional central access obtained as needed. If the peritoneum is breached in a peritoneal dialysis patient, alternative access for dialysis needs to be considered as peritoneal dialysis is less likely to be successful.

Depending on the immunological risk of the patient, in the presence of DGF, a reduction in target tacrolimus levels can be contemplated. Many transplant centres target a tacrolimus level 8–10 μg/L in the peri-transplantation period. Provided the patient is not considered high immunological risk, reduction of the target range could be considered. The use of thymoglobulin in the setting of DGF is controversial in the absence of immunological risk factors advocating its use as an induction agent [15].

Risk factor	Relative impact
Donation after circulatory death	2× higher rate of ATN. No difference in outcome at 1 year
Donor on inotropes	Early function 58% (vs. 83%). 1-year survival 73% (vs. 91%)
Cold ischemia time	23% increase risk of DGF for every 6 h
Donor age > 55y	2× higher rate of DGF
Other donor factors	Poor reperfusion, death from stroke, presence of AKI associated with increased risk
Higher PRA%	Associated higher risk of requiring dialysis post-transplant
Recipient hypovolaemia	Lower pre-operative DBP, intra-operative albumin requirement and pre-operative haemodialysis with UF
Dialysis modality	Higher rate of DGF in haemodialysis vs. peritoneal dialysis
Special circumstances	Thrombophilia, previous transplant

Adapted from Perico et al. [75].

Table 8.
Risk factors for delayed graft function.

5.5 Renal vascular complication

In transplant recipients who have established a good urine output post-operatively, the sudden development of oliguria or anuria should prompt a review of urinary catheter patency as well as raise the possibility of transplant vessel pathology. Early vascular pathology may be caused by structural or anatomical factors such as vessel kinking, anatomically disadvantageous configurations putting traction on the recipient vessels or thrombosis. Distinguishing between the various pathologies can be challenging clinically, with reliance on duplex ultrasound imaging and knowledge of donor vascular pathology through collaboration with transplant surgeons.

Renal transplant artery or vein thrombosis is a serious, although fortunately uncommon peri-transplant complication, with an incidence of 2–3%, classically occurring in the first week post-transplant [77]. Clinical features of transplant artery thrombosis are typically limited to the sudden onset of oligoanuria, while transplant vein thrombosis may cause allograft swelling, pain and frank haematuria in addition. Predisposing risk factors are decreased perfusion pressures and hypotension as well as donor factors—difficult bench surgery, multiple vessels, prolonged cold ischaemia time and vessel atherosclerosis [77, 88]. Rarer recipient risk factors, when present, can dramatically increase the risk of thrombosis, including in the transplant vessels. Recipients with thrombophilia, notably factor V Leiden mutation or anti-phospholipid antibodies, have been associated with higher risk (2.87 increased risk in one study) of adverse graft outcomes [89, 90]. Diagnosis of transplant vessel pathology may be obtained by urgent renal duplex ultrasonography; however, the abrupt onset of anuria in the early post-operative period is an indication for urgent surgical review and consideration of surgical re-exploration, due to the very short window after transplant arterial thrombosis before irretrievable graft loss occurs.

Renal transplant artery stenosis tends to be a later complication but can occasionally manifest in the perioperative period. The classical clinical features associated with stenosis of the transplant artery are hypertension, allograft dysfunction and fluid overload due to salt and water retention. Risk factors for early transplant artery stenosis tend to be donor related with atherosclerotic vessels or difficult bench surgery [77]. An association with acute rejection has also been described [91]. Diagnosis is by duplex scan showing increased velocity across the anastomotic sites and a flow differential between the aorta and transplant artery.

Intermittent vessel kinking caused by allograft nephroptosis can be diagnostically challenging due to the positional nature of the pathology [92]. Duplex scans may be non-diagnostic, and performing imaging in a non-prone position may assist in the diagnosis of positional vessel compression or kinking, and CT angiography may provide additional diagnostic information in this situation.

5.6 Renal ureteric complications

Ureteric pathology is more common than vascular pathology, but rarely affects graft survival [93]. The most common early urological complication is a urine leak with an estimated incidence of 8%, followed by ureteric stenoses with a similar incidence occurring later in the transplant course [77, 94]. Other complications of vesicoureteric reflux and urolithiasis are uncommon [95].

Ureteric leaks, like vascular pathology, typically occur in first few weeks post-transplant and may present with localised pain or swelling at the site of the allograft, increased surgical drain output or a peri-transplant collection seen on imaging [95]. Non-technical risk factors include recipient agent, pre-transplant urological pathology, immunosuppressive regimen and donor factors [94].

When there is a clinical suspicion for a urine leak due to increased surgical drain output, or if a peri-transplant collection is drained, the fluid should be sent for creatinine concentration analysis to differentiate serous or lymphatic fluid (which will have a similar creatinine concentration to the blood) from urine. Following drain removal, recipients with a urine leak may complain of pain due to fluid accumulation or if there is a significant urine leak, graft function will appear to deteriorate due to reabsorption of urinary creatinine and urea.

The management of urine leaks can be complex and often requires liaison with a transplant urologist. It may be possible to manage minor urine leaks conservatively via bladder decompression with an indwelling catheter in addition to ureteric stenting to allow the distal anastomosis to heal. Larger leaks may require further investigation in contrast to enhanced computer tomography, insertion of a percutaneous nephrostomy or surgical repair [95]. A more detailed discussion of this topic is beyond the scope of this chapter.

5.7 Infection

As a consequence of induction immunosuppression, transplant patients are particularly prone to infection in the perioperative phase. However, sepsis can be challenging to diagnose during this period because immunocompromised patients may not manifest the typical features of a systemic inflammatory response. Due to steroid therapy, most patients will exhibit a peripheral neutrophilia. In general, any change in physiological parameters, clinical deterioration or a temperature > 37.5°C should prompt consideration of sepsis, and a sepsis screen should be requested including [96]:

- haematology panel
- C-reactive protein
- blood culture and venous lactate
- urinalysis and urine culture
- chest X-ray
- additional testing as appropriate—respiratory virus screen, lumbar puncture, opportunistic infection screen
- empiric antibiotic therapy within 1 h of suspected sepsis diagnosis

Although transplant recipients are susceptible to opportunistic pathogens such as CMV, EBV, mycobacteria, *Pneumocystis jiroveci* and fungi, these are unusual in the early post-transplant period. Infections occurring soon after transplantation are frequently nosocomial, associated with hospitalisation, intravenous and urinary catheters and intubation during surgery. In some instances, infection may be donor derived [97].

5.7.1 Bacterial infection

Urinary tract infections (UTI) are the most common cause of bacterial infection requiring hospitalisation in transplant patients, followed by pneumonia, surgical site infections and septicaemia [98]. Retrospective database studies have estimated a cumulative incidence of 17% in the first 6 months post-transplant, which rises to 60% for women and 47% for men at 3 years [99]. The presentation for UTI is similar to that of the general population and management identical to complicated UTIs with 7–14 days of antibiotic therapy, although the optimal duration has not been well established [98]. Management of post-transplant candiduria is controversial, without definite improvement in clinical outcomes following therapy [100]. Other bacterial pathologies are treated in the same way as in the general population with anticipated more frequent and longer duration antibiotic use due to physician concern over immunosuppressed state and propensity for more severe infection.

5.8 Rejection

In the early era of transplantation, hyperacute rejection due to the presence of preformed donor-specific antibodies (DSAs) occurring in the first minutes or hours after perfusion of the transplant was a significant risk. However, with the introduction of the complement-dependent cytotoxic cross-match, as described by Patel and Terasaki [101], and more recently solid phase assays that are able to detect DSAs with high sensitivity, hyperacute rejection is now extremely rare [102]. Nevertheless, early acute rejection remains a common occurrence, with a reported incidence of 7–25% depending on the level of immunological risk and choice of induction immunosuppression [21, 103–106]. Contemporary rejection rates in Australia and New Zealand are shown in **Table 9**.

In the perioperative period, DGF persisting beyond 4–5 days, decreasing urine output or an unexplained rise in creatinine by >15–20%, should prompt consideration of rejection as the underlying cause (Section 5.4). Unless there is a contraindication such as active bleeding or an unavoidable requirement for anticoagulation, the diagnosis requires a renal biopsy, both to exclude alternative causes of graft dysfunction and to characterise the histological pattern and severity of rejection. Rejection is classified histologically using the Banff criteria into borderline rejection, cell-mediated rejection, antibody-mediated rejection and mixed rejection [107, 108]. Treatment of cellular rejection would usually involve pulsed methylprednisolone 0.25–1.0 g daily for 3 days as first-line treatment, combined with a T-cell depleting therapy such as thymoglobulin/ATG if the rejection is histologically severe rejection (Banff class 2 or greater), or if there is a suboptimal response to methylprednisolone [109]. The optimal therapy for acute antibody-mediated rejection remains unclear, but would typically include pulsed methylprednisolone, plasma exchange (often combined with intravenous immunoglobulin at a dose of 0.1 g/kg following each exchange) outcomes [110–112]. Some centres also advocate the use of a B cell depleting antibody such as rituximab or the proteasome inhibitor bortezomib, although currently there is no strong evidence that these agents improve clinical outcomes [111, 113–115].

	First allograft (%)	Second or subsequent allograft (%)
Living donor	17.4	16.7
Deceased donor	15.2	18.6

Data from ANZDATA Registry. 41st Report, Chapter 7: Kidney Transplantation. Australia and New Zealand Dialysis and Transplant Registry, Adelaide, Australia. 2018. http://www.anzdata.org.au.

Table 9.
Acute rejection rates in the first six months post-transplant.

6. Conclusions

Kidney transplantation has evolved from a highly experimental therapy to become recognised as the gold standard treatment for many patients with ESKD [116]. This progress has occurred through the many iterative developments in the surgical and medical management of transplant recipients, not the least of which being the introduction of highly effective immunosuppressive agents. Delivering high standards of clinical care during the perioperative period is a crucial step in achieving excellent allograft outcomes. This chapter provides an overview of the approach to assessing potential recipients admitted for transplantation, and guidance on typical perioperative medication and fluid prescriptions, as well as post-operative monitoring and early complications.

Conflict of interest

David Johnson has previously received consultancy fees, research grants, speaker's honoraria and travel sponsorships from Baxter Healthcare and Fresenius Medical Care. He has also received consultancy fees from Astra Zeneca and travel sponsorships from Amgen. He is a current recipient of an Australian National Health and Medical Research Council Practitioner Fellowship. Carmel Hawley has received a research grant from Baxter Healthcare. Ross Francis has received honoraria and travel sponsorships from Novartis, Astellas and Amgen. The other authors have no conflict of interest to declare.

Notes/thanks/other declarations

Nil.

Author details

Sebastian Hultin[1], Carmel M. Hawley[1,2,3], David W. Johnson[1,2,3] and Ross S. Francis[1*]

1 Department of Nephrology, Princess Alexandra Hospital, Brisbane, Australia

2 Australasian Kidney Trials Network, Centre for Health Services Research, University of Queensland, Brisbane, Australia

3 Translational Research Unit, Brisbane, Australia

*Address all correspondence to: ross.francis@health.qld.gov.au

References

[1] Jha V, Modi GK. Getting to know the enemy better-the global burden of chronic kidney disease. Kidney International. 2018;**94**(3):462-464

[2] Xie Y, Bowe B, Mokdad AH, Xian H, Yan Y, Li T, et al. Analysis of the Global Burden of Disease study highlights the global, regional, and national trends of chronic kidney disease epidemiology from 1990 to 2016. Kidney International. 2018;**94**(3):567-581

[3] Collins AJ, Foley RN, Herzog C, Chavers BM, Gilbertson D, Ishani A, et al. Excerpts from the US Renal Data System 2009 Annual Data Report. American Journal of Kidney Diseases: The Official Journal of the National Kidney Foundation. 2010;**55**(1 Suppl 1):S1-S420, a6-7

[4] Tonelli M, Wiebe N, Knoll G, Bello A, Browne S, Jadhav D, et al. Systematic review: Kidney transplantation compared with dialysis in clinically relevant outcomes. American Journal of Transplantation: Official Journal of the American Society of Transplantation and the American Society of Transplant Surgeons. 2011;**11**(10):2093-2109

[5] McDonald SP, Russ GR. Survival of recipients of cadaveric kidney transplants compared with those receiving dialysis treatment in Australia and New Zealand, 1991-2001. Nephrology, Dialysis, Transplantation: Official Publication of the European Dialysis and Transplant Association-European Renal Association. 2002;**17**(12):2212-2219

[6] Evenepoel P, Van Den Bergh B, Naesens M, De Jonge H, Bammens B, Claes K, et al. Calcium metabolism in the early posttransplantation period. Clinical Journal of the American Society of Nephrology: CJASN. 2009;**4**(3):665-672

[7] London MJ. Perioperative beta-blockade, discontinuation, and complications: Do you really know it when you see it? Anesthesiology. 2009;**111**(4):690-694

[8] Yang BR, Seong JM, Choi NK, Shin JY, Lee J, Kim YJ, et al. Co-medication of statins with contraindicated drugs. PLoS One. 2015;**10**(5):e0125180

[9] Robertson AJ, Nargund V, Gray DW, Morris PJ. Low dose aspirin as prophylaxis against renal-vein thrombosis in renal-transplant recipients. Nephrology, Dialysis, Transplantation. 2000;**15**(11):1865-1868

[10] Molnar MZ, Czira M, Ambrus C, Szeifert L, Szentkiralyi A, Beko G, et al. Anemia is associated with mortality in kidney-transplanted patients—A prospective cohort study. American Journal of Transplantation: Official Journal of the American Society of Transplantation and the American Society of Transplant Surgeons. 2007;**7**(4):818-824

[11] KDIGO clinical practice guideline for the care of kidney transplant recipients. American Journal of Transplantation: Official Journal of the American Society of Transplantation and the American Society of Transplant Surgeons. 2009;**9**(Suppl 3):S1-S155

[12] Locatelli F, Aljama P, Barany P, Canaud B, Carrera F, Eckardt KU, et al. Revised European best practice guidelines for the management of anaemia in patients with chronic renal failure. Nephrology, Dialysis, Transplantation: Official Publication of the European Dialysis and Transplant Association—European Renal Association. 2004;**19**(Suppl 2):ii1-47

[13] Tran HA, Chunilal SD, Tran H. An update of consensus guidelines for

warfarin reversal. The Medical Journal of Australia. 2014;**200**(2):82

[14] Webster AC, Ruster LP, McGee R, Matheson SL, Higgins GY, Willis NS, et al. Interleukin 2 receptor antagonists for kidney transplant recipients. Cochrane Database of Systematic Reviews. 2010;**1**:CD003897

[15] Brennan DC, Daller JA, Lake KD, Cibrik D, Del Castillo D, Group ftTIS. Rabbit antithymocyte globulin versus basiliximab in renal transplantation. The New England Journal of Medicine. 2006;**355**:1967-1977

[16] 3C Study Collaborative Group. Alemtuzumab-based induction treatment versus basiliximab-based induction treatment in kidney transplantation (the 3C Study): A randomised trial. The Lancet. 2014. [Epub ahead of print]

[17] Morgan RD, O'Callaghan JM, Knight SR, Morris PJ. Alemtuzumab induction therapy in kidney transplantation: A systematic review and meta-analysis. Transplantation. 2012;**93**(12):1179-1188

[18] Morris PJ, Russell NK. Alemtuzumab (Campath-1H): A systematic review in organ transplantation. Transplantation. 2006;**81**(10):1361-1367

[19] Halloran PF. Immunosuppressive drugs for kidney transplantation. The New England Journal of Medicine. 2004;**351**(26):2715-2729

[20] Opelz G, Dohler B. Influence of immunosuppressive regimens on graft survival and secondary outcomes after kidney transplantation. Transplantation. 2009;**87**(6):795-802

[21] Ekberg H, Tedesco-Silva H, Demirbas A, Vitko S, Nashan B, Gurkan A, et al. Reduced exposure to calcineurin inhibitors in renal transplantation. The New England Journal of Medicine. 2007;**357**(25):2562-2575

[22] Batiuk TD, Bodziak KA, Goldman M. Infectious disease prophylaxis in renal transplant patients: A survey of US transplant centers. Clinical Transplantation. 2002;**16**(1):1-8

[23] Orlando G, Manzia TM, Sorge R, Iaria G, Angelico R, Sforza D, et al. One-shot versus multidose perioperative antibiotic prophylaxis after kidney transplantation: A randomized, controlled clinical trial. Surgery. 2015;**157**(1):104-110

[24] Chan SNS, Chan HP, Pascoe E, Playford E, Wong G, Chapman JR, et al. Perioperative antibiotics for preventing post-surgical site infections in solid organ transplant recipients. Cochrane Database of Systematic Reviews. 2018;(12)

[25] Martin SI, Fishman JA, Practice ASTIDCo. Pneumocystis pneumonia in solid organ transplantation. American Journal of Transplantation. 2013;**13**(Suppl 4):272-279

[26] Gordon SM, LaRosa SP, Kalmadi S, Arroliga AC, Avery RK, Truesdell-LaRosa L, et al. Should prophylaxis for Pneumocystis carinii pneumonia in solid organ transplant recipients ever be discontinued? Clinical Infectious Diseases: An Official Publication of the Infectious Diseases Society of America. 1999;**28**(2):240-246

[27] Chapman JR, Marriott DJ, Chen SC, MacDonald PS. Post-transplant Pneumocystis jirovecii pneumonia—A re-emerged public health problem? Kidney International. 2013;**84**(2):240-243

[28] Playford EG, Webster AC, Sorell TC, Craig JC. Antifungal agents for preventing fungal infections in solid organ transplant recipients. Cochrane

Database of Systematic Reviews. 2004;**3**:CD004291

[29] Guerra CM, Formica RN, Kulkarni S, Asch WS, Tichy EM. Duration of prophylaxis against fungal infection in kidney transplant recipients. Progress in Transplantation (Aliso Viejo, Calif). 2015;**25**(4):311-315

[30] Fishman JA, Emery V, Freeman R, Pascual M, Rostaing L, Schlitt HJ, et al. Cytomegalovirus in transplantation—Challenging the status quo. Clinical Transplantation. 2007;**21**(2):149-158

[31] Hodson EM, Ladhani M, Webster AC, Strippoli GF, Craig JC. Antiviral medications for preventing cytomegalovirus disease in solid organ transplant recipients. The Cochrane Database of Systematic Reviews. 2013;(2):Cd003774

[32] Hodson EM, Craig JC, Strippoli GF, Webster AC. Antiviral medications for preventing cytomegalovirus disease in solid organ transplant recipients. The Cochrane Database of Systematic Reviews. 2008;(2):Cd003774

[33] AlDabbagh MA, Gitman MR, Kumar D, Humar A, Rotstein C, Husain S. The role of antiviral prophylaxis for the prevention of Epstein-Barr virus-associated posttransplant lymphoproliferative disease in solid organ transplant recipients: A systematic review. American Journal of Transplantation. 2017;**17**(3):770-781

[34] Luan FL, Stuckey LJ, Park JM, Kaul D, Cibrik D, Ojo A. Six-month prophylaxis is cost effective in transplant patients at high risk for cytomegalovirus infection. Journal of the American Society of Nephrology: JASN. 2009;**20**(11):2449-2458

[35] Owers DS, Webster AC, Strippoli GF, Kable K, Hodson EM. Pre-emptive treatment for cytomegalovirus viraemia to prevent cytomegalovirus disease in solid organ transplant recipients. The Cochrane Database of Systematic Reviews. 2013;(2):Cd005133

[36] Ray S, Delaney M, Muller AF. Proton pump inhibitors and acute interstitial nephritis. BMJ (Clinical Research Ed). 2010;**341**:c4412

[37] Rodriguez-Poncelas A, Barcelo MA, Saez M, Coll-de-Tuero G. Duration and dosing of Proton Pump Inhibitors associated with high incidence of chronic kidney disease in population-based cohort. PLoS One. 2018;**13**(10):e0204231

[38] Gould MK, Garcia DA, Wren SM, Karanicolas PJ, Arcelus JI, Heit JA, et al. Prevention of VTE in nonorthopedic surgical patients: Antithrombotic Therapy and Prevention of Thrombosis, 9th ed: American College of Chest Physicians Evidence-Based Clinical Practice Guidelines. Chest. 2012;**141**(2 Suppl):e227S-ee77S

[39] Jun KW, Park KM, Kim MH, Hwang JK, Park SC, Moon IS, et al. Mechanical thromboprophylaxis is sufficient to prevent the lower extremity deep vein thrombosis after kidney transplantation. Annals of Surgical Treatment and Research. 2014;**87**(1):28-34

[40] Lemmens HJ. Kidney transplantation: Recent developments and recommendations for anesthetic management. Anesthesiology Clinics of North America. 2004;**22**(4):651-662

[41] Othman MM, Ismael AZ, Hammouda GE. The impact of timing of maximal crystalloid hydration on early graft function during kidney transplantation. Anesthesia and Analgesia. 2010;**110**(5):1440-1446

[42] Campos L, Parada B, Furriel F, Castelo D, Moreira P, Mota A. Do intraoperative hemodynamic factors of the recipient influence renal graft function? Transplantation Proceedings. 2012;**44**(6):1800-1803

[43] Marik PE, Cavallazzi R. Does the central venous pressure predict fluid responsiveness? An updated meta-analysis and a plea for some common sense. Critical Care Medicine. 2013;**41**(7):1774-1781

[44] Brienza N, Giglio MT, Marucci M, Fiore T. Does perioperative hemodynamic optimization protect renal function in surgical patients? A meta-analytic study. Critical Care Medicine. 2009;**37**(6):2079-2090

[45] Myles PS, Bellomo R, Corcoran T, Forbes A, Peyton P, Story D, et al. Restrictive versus liberal fluid therapy for major abdominal surgery. The New England Journal of Medicine. 2018;**378**(24):2263-2274

[46] Weimar W, Geerlings W, Bijnen AB, Obertop H, van Urk H, Lameijer LD, et al. A controlled study on the effect of mannitol on immediate renal function after cadaver donor kidney transplantation. Transplantation. 1983;**35**(1):99-101

[47] Calixto Fernandes MH, Schricker T, Magder S, Hatzakorzian R. Perioperative fluid management in kidney transplantation: A black box. Critical Care (London, England). 2018;**22**(1):14

[48] Naesens M, Heylen L, Lerut E, Claes K, De Wever L, Claus F, et al. Intrarenal resistive index after renal transplantation. The New England Journal of Medicine. 2013;**369**(19):1797-1806

[49] Benjamens S, Pol RA, de Geus-Oei LF, de Vries APJ, Glaudemans A, Berger SP, et al. Can transplant renal scintigraphy predict the duration of delayed graft function? A dual center retrospective study. PLoS One. 2018;**13**(3):e0193791

[50] El-Maghraby TA, Boom H, Camps JA, Blokland KA, Zwinderman AH, Paul LC, et al. Delayed graft function is characterized by reduced functional mass measured by (99m)Technetium-mercaptoacetyltriglycine renography. Transplantation. 2002;**74**(2):203-208

[51] Van Laecke S, Van Biesen W, Verbeke F, De Bacquer D, Peeters P, Vanholder R. Posttransplantation hypomagnesemia and its relation with immunosuppression as predictors of new-onset diabetes after transplantation. American Journal of Transplantation. 2009;**9**(9):2140-2149

[52] Kaiser W. Cyclosporin treatment and hypomagnesaemia. Nephrology, Dialysis, Transplantation. 1992;**7**(12):1257-1258

[53] Baia LC, Heilberg IP, Navis G, de Borst MH, NIGRAM Investigators. Phosphate and FGF-23 homeostasis after kidney transplantation. Nature Reviews. Nephrology. 2015;**11**(11):656-666

[54] Seeherunvong W, Wolf M. Tertiary excess of fibroblast growth factor 23 and hypophosphatemia following kidney transplantation. Pediatric Transplantation. 2011;**15**(1):37-46

[55] Yang Y, Yu B, Chen Y. Blood disorders typically associated with renal transplantation. Frontiers in Cell and Developmental Biology. 2015;**3**:18

[56] Mathew TH. A blinded, long-term, randomized multicenter study of mycophenolate mofetil in cadaveric renal transplantation: Results at three years. Tricontinental Mycophenolate Mofetil Renal Transplantation Study Group. Transplantation. 1998;**65**(11):1450-1454

[57] Webster AC, Lee VW, Chapman JR, Craig JC. Target of rapamycin inhibitors (TOR-I; sirolimus and everolimus) for primary immunosuppression in kidney transplant recipients. The Cochrane Database of Systematic Reviews. 2006;(2):Cd004290

[58] Paya C, Humar A, Dominguez E, Washburn K, Blumberg E, Alexander B, et al. Efficacy and safety of valganciclovir vs. oral ganciclovir for prevention of cytomegalovirus disease in solid organ transplant recipients. American Journal of Transplantation: Official Journal of the American Society of Transplantation and the American Society of Transplant Surgeons. 2004;**4**(4):611-620

[59] Ozer H, Armitage JO, Bennett CL, Crawford J, Demetri GD, Pizzo PA, et al. 2000 update of recommendations for the use of hematopoietic colony-stimulating factors: Evidence-based, clinical practice guidelines. American Society of Clinical Oncology Growth Factors Expert Panel. Journal of Clinical Oncology: Official Journal of the American Society of Clinical Oncology. 2000;**18**(20):3558-3585

[60] Eid AJ, Chen SF, Practice ASTIDCo. Human parvovirus B19 in solid organ transplantation. American Journal of Transplantation. 2013;**13**(Suppl 4):201-205

[61] Warner MA, Woodrum D, Hanson A, Schroeder DR, Wilson G, Kor DJ. Preprocedural platelet transfusion for patients with thrombocytopenia undergoing interventional radiology procedures is not associated with reduced bleeding complications. Transfusion. 2017;**57**(4):890-898

[62] Mundra VRR, Mannon RB. Thrombotic microangiopathy in a transplant recipient. Clinical Journal of the American Society of Nephrology. 2018;**13**(8):1251-1253

[63] Chiurchiu C, Ruggenenti P, Remuzzi G. Thrombotic microangiopathy in renal transplantation. Annals of Transplantation. 2002;**7**(1):28-33

[64] Ponticelli C. De novo thrombotic microangiopathy. An underrated complication of renal transplantation. Clinical Nephrology. 2007;**67**(6):335-340

[65] Zuber J, Le Quintrec M, Sberro-Soussan R, Loirat C, Fremeaux-Bacchi V, Legendre C. New insights into postrenal transplant hemolytic uremic syndrome. Nature Reviews. Nephrology. 2011;**7**(1):23-35

[66] Fox LC, Cohney SJ, Kausman JY, Shortt J, Hughes PD, Wood EM, et al. Consensus opinion on diagnosis and management of thrombotic microangiopathy in Australia and New Zealand. Nephrology (Carlton, Vic.). 2018;**23**(6):507-517

[67] Hecking M, Werzowa J, Haidinger M, Horl WH, Pascual J, Budde K, et al. Novel views on new-onset diabetes after transplantation: Development, prevention and treatment. Nephrology, Dialysis, Transplantation. 2013;**28**(3):550-566

[68] Chakkera HA, Knowler WC, Devarapalli Y, Weil EJ, Heilman RL, Dueck A, et al. Relationship between inpatient hyperglycemia and insulin treatment after kidney transplantation and future new onset diabetes mellitus. Clinical Journal of the American Society of Nephrology. 2010;**5**(9):1669-1675

[69] Cosio FG, Kudva Y, van der Velde M, Larson TS, Textor SC, Griffin MD, et al. New onset hyperglycemia and diabetes are associated with increased cardiovascular risk after kidney transplantation. Kidney International. 2005;**67**(6):2415-2421

[70] Mourad G, Glyda M, Albano L, Viklicky O, Merville P, Tyden G, et al. Incidence of posttransplantation diabetes mellitus in de novo kidney transplant recipients receiving prolonged-release tacrolimus-based immunosuppression with 2 different corticosteroid minimization strategies: ADVANCE, a randomized controlled trial. Transplantation. 2017;**101**(8):1924-1934

[71] Yates CJ, Fourlanos S, Colman PG, Cohney SJ. Screening for new-onset diabetes after kidney transplantation: Limitations of fasting glucose and advantages of afternoon glucose and glycated hemoglobin. Transplantation. 2013;**96**(8):726-731

[72] First MR, Dhadda S, Croy R, Holman J, Fitzsimmons WE. New-onset diabetes after transplantation (NODAT): An evaluation of definitions in clinical trials. Transplantation. 2013;**96**(1):58-64

[73] Yates CJ, Fourlanos S, Hjelmesaeth J, Colman PG, Cohney SJ. New-onset diabetes after kidney transplantation-changes and challenges. American Journal of Transplantation. 2012;**12**(4):820-828

[74] Thomas MC, Moran J, Mathew TH, Russ GR, Rao MM. Early perioperative hyperglycaemia and renal allograft rejection in patients without diabetes. BMC Nephrology. 2000;**1**:1

[75] Perico N, Cattaneo D, Sayegh MH, Remuzzi G. Delayed graft function in kidney transplantation. Lancet (London, England). 2004;**364**(9447):1814-1827

[76] Dawidson IJ, Sandor ZF, Coorpender L, Palmer B, Peters P, Lu C, et al. Intraoperative albumin administration affects the outcome of cadaver renal transplantation. Transplantation. 1992;**53**(4):774-782

[77] Hernandez D, Rufino M, Armas S, Gonzalez A, Gutierrez P, Barbero P, et al. Retrospective analysis of surgical complications following cadaveric kidney transplantation in the modern transplant era. Nephrology, Dialysis, Transplantation: Official Publication of the European Dialysis and Transplant Association—European Renal Association. 2006;**21**(10):2908-2915

[78] Ferrandiz I, Congy-Jolivet N, Del Bello A, Debiol B, Trebern-Launay K, Esposito L, et al. Impact of early blood transfusion after kidney transplantation on the incidence of donor-specific anti-HLA antibodies. American Journal of Transplantation. 2016;**16**(9):2661-2669

[79] Foley RN, Parfrey PS, Harnett JD, Kent GM, Murray DC, Barre PE. Hypoalbuminemia, cardiac morbidity, and mortality in end-stage renal disease. Journal of the American Society of Nephrology: JASN. 1996;**7**(5):728-736

[80] Humar A, Kerr SR, Ramcharan T, Gillingham KJ, Matas AJ. Perioperative cardiac morbidity in kidney transplant recipients: Incidence and risk factors. Clinical Transplantation. 2001;**15**(3):154-158

[81] Hoorn EJ, Walsh SB, McCormick JA, Furstenberg A, Yang CL, Roeschel T, et al. The calcineurin inhibitor tacrolimus activates the renal sodium chloride cotransporter to cause hypertension. Nature Medicine. 2011;**17**(10):1304-1309

[82] Wang LW, Fahim MA, Hayen A, Mitchell RL, Baines L, Lord S, et al. Cardiac testing for coronary artery disease in potential kidney transplant recipients. The Cochrane Database of Systematic Reviews. 2011;(12):Cd008691

[83] Herzog CA, Marwick TH, Pheley AM, White CW, Rao VK, Dick CD. Dobutamine stress echocardiography for the detection of significant coronary artery disease in renal transplant candidates. American Journal of Kidney Diseases: The Official Journal of the National Kidney Foundation. 1999;**33**(6):1080-1090

[84] Stidley CA, Hunt WC, Tentori F, Schmidt D, Rohrscheib M, Paine S, et al. Changing relationship of blood pressure with mortality over time among

hemodialysis patients. Journal of the American Society of Nephrology: JASN. 2006;**17**(2):513-520

[85] Wheeler DC, Becker GJ. Summary of KDIGO guideline. What do we really know about management of blood pressure in patients with chronic kidney disease? Kidney International. 2013;**83**(3):377-383

[86] Lim WH, Johnson DW, Teixeira-Pinto A, Wong G. Association between duration of delayed graft function, acute rejection and allograft outcome after deceased donor kidney transplantation. Transplantation. 2018

[87] Yarlagadda SG, Coca SG, Formica RN Jr, Poggio ED, Parikh CR. Association between delayed graft function and allograft and patient survival: A systematic review and meta-analysis. Nephrology, Dialysis, Transplantation: Official Publication of the European Dialysis and Transplant Association—European Renal Association. 2009;**24**(3):1039-1047

[88] Bakir N, Sluiter WJ, Ploeg RJ, van Son WJ, Tegzess AM. Primary renal graft thrombosis. Nephrology, Dialysis, Transplantation: Official Publication of the European Dialysis and Transplant Association—European Renal Association. 1996;**11**(1):140-147

[89] Wagenknecht DR, Becker DG, LeFor WM, McIntyre JA. Antiphospholipid antibodies are a risk factor for early renal allograft failure. Transplantation. 1999;**68**(2):241-246

[90] Hocher B, Slowinski T, Hauser I, Vetter B, Fritsche L, Bachert D, et al. Association of factor V Leiden mutation with delayed graft function, acute rejection episodes and long-term graft dysfunction in kidney transplant recipients. Thrombosis and Haemostasis. 2002;**87**(2):194-198

[91] Buturovic-Ponikvar J. Renal transplant artery stenosis. Nephrology, Dialysis, Transplantation: Official Publication of the European Dialysis and Transplant Association—European Renal Association. 2003;**18**(Suppl 5):v74-v77

[92] Dosch AR, Pahl M, Reddy U, Foster CE 3rd, Ichii H. Post-transplantation nephroptosis causing recurrent episodes of acute renal failure and hypertension secondary to intermittent vascular torsion of intraperitoneal renal allograft. Journal of Surgical Case Reports. 2017;**2017**(5):rjx033

[93] van Roijen JH, Kirkels WJ, Zietse R, Roodnat JI, Weimar W, Ijzermans JN. Long-term graft survival after urological complications of 695 kidney transplantations. The Journal of Urology. 2001;**165**(6 Pt 1):1884-1887

[94] Rodriguez Faba O, Boissier R, Budde K, Figueiredo A, Taylor CF, Hevia V, et al. European association of urology guidelines on renal transplantation: Update 2018. European Urology Focus. 2018;**4**(2):208-215

[95] Branchereau J, Karam G. Management of urologic complications of renal transplantation. European Urology Supplements. 2016;**15**(9):408-414

[96] Rhodes A, Evans LE, Alhazzani W, Levy MM, Antonelli M, Ferrer R, et al. Surviving sepsis campaign: International guidelines for management of sepsis and septic shock: 2016. Intensive Care Medicine. 2017;**43**(3):304-377

[97] White SL, Rawlinson W, Boan P, Sheppeard V, Wong G, Waller K, et al. Infectious disease transmission in solid organ transplantation. Donor Evaluation, Recipient Risk, and Outcomes of Transmission. Transplantation Direct. 2019;**5**(1):e416

[98] Karuthu S, Blumberg EA. Common infections in kidney transplant recipients. Clinical Journal of the American Society of Nephrology: CJASN. 2012;**7**(12):2058-2070

[99] Abbott KC, Swanson SJ, Richter ER, Bohen EM, Agodoa LY, Peters TG, et al. Late urinary tract infection after renal transplantation in the United States. American Journal of Kidney Diseases: The Official Journal of the National Kidney Foundation. 2004;**44**(2):353-362

[100] Safdar N, Slattery WR, Knasinski V, Gangnon RE, Li Z, Pirsch JD, et al. Predictors and outcomes of candiduria in renal transplant recipients. Clinical Infectious Diseases: An Official Publication of the Infectious Diseases Society of America. 2005;**40**(10):1413-1421

[101] Patel R, Terasaki PI. Significance of the positive crossmatch test in kidney transplantation. The New England Journal of Medicine. 1969;**280**(14):735-739

[102] Zhang R. Donor-specific antibodies in kidney transplant recipients. Clinical Journal of the American Society of Nephrology. 2018;**13**(1):182-192

[103] Wu WK, Famure O, Li Y, Kim SJ. Delayed graft function and the risk of acute rejection in the modern era of kidney transplantation. Kidney International. 2015;**88**(4):851-858

[104] Pascual J, Berger SP, Witzke O, Tedesco H, Mulgaonkar S, Qazi Y, et al. Everolimus with reduced calcineurin inhibitor exposure in renal transplantation. Journal of the American Society of Nephrology. 2018;**29**(7):1979-1991

[105] Group CSC, Haynes R, Harden P, Judge P, Blackwell L, Emberson J, et al. Alemtuzumab-based induction treatment versus basiliximab-based induction treatment in kidney transplantation (the 3C Study): A randomised trial. Lancet. 2014;**384**(9955):1684-1690

[106] Tanriover B, Jaikaransingh V, MacConmara MP, Parekh JR, Levea SL, Ariyamuthu VK, et al. Acute rejection rates and graft outcomes according to induction regimen among recipients of kidneys from deceased donors treated with tacrolimus and mycophenolate. Clinical Journal of the American Society of Nephrology. 2016;**11**(9):1650-1661

[107] Haas M, Loupy A, Lefaucheur C, Roufosse C, Glotz D, Seron D, et al. The Banff 2017 Kidney Meeting Report: Revised diagnostic criteria for chronic active T cell-mediated rejection, antibody-mediated rejection, and prospects for integrative endpoints for next-generation clinical trials. American Journal of Transplantation: Official Journal of the American Society of Transplantation and the American Society of Transplant Surgeons. 2018;**18**(2):293-307

[108] Roufosse C, Simmonds N, Clahsen-van Groningen M, Haas M, Henriksen KJ, Horsfield C, et al. A 2018 reference guide to the Banff classification of renal allograft pathology. Transplantation. 2018;**102**(11):1795-1814

[109] Webster AC, Wu S, Tallapragada K, Park MY, Chapman JR, Carr SJ. Polyclonal and monoclonal antibodies for treating acute rejection episodes in kidney transplant recipients. The Cochrane Database of Systematic Reviews. 2017;**7**:Cd004756

[110] Lefaucheur C, Loupy A. Antibody-mediated rejection of solid-organ allografts. The New England Journal of Medicine. 2018;**379**(26):2580-2582

[111] Wan SS, Ying TD, Wyburn K, Roberts DM, Wyld M, Chadban SJ. The treatment of antibody-mediated rejection in kidney transplantation: An updated systematic review and

meta-analysis. Transplantation. 2018;**102**(4):557-568

[112] Velidedeoglu E, Cavaille-Coll MW, Bala S, Belen OA, Wang Y, Albrecht R. Summary of 2017 FDA Public Workshop: Antibody-mediated rejection in kidney transplantation. Transplantation. 2018;**102**(6):e257-ee64

[113] Eskandary F, Regele H, Baumann L, Bond G, Kozakowski N, Wahrmann M, et al. A randomized trial of bortezomib in late antibody-mediated kidney transplant rejection. Journal of the American Society of Nephrology. 2018;**29**(2):591-605

[114] Sautenet B, Blancho G, Buchler M, Morelon E, Toupance O, Barrou B, et al. One-year results of the effects of rituximab on acute antibody-mediated rejection in renal transplantation: RITUX ERAH, a multicenter double-blind randomized placebo-controlled trial. Transplantation. 2016;**100**(2):391-399

[115] Becker YT, Becker BN, Pirsch JD, Sollinger HW. Rituximab as treatment for refractory kidney transplant rejection. American Journal of Transplantation. 2004;**4**(6):996-1001

[116] Morris PJ. Transplantation—A medical miracle of the 20th century. The New England Journal of Medicine. 2004;**351**(26):2678-2680

Chapter 3

Viral Infections after Kidney Transplantation: CMV and BK

Večerić-Haler Željka and Kojc Nika

Abstract

Opportunistic infections commonly occur during the first 6 months after kidney transplant, including cytomegalovirus (CMV) and polyomaviruses. Viral pathogens such as CMV and polyomaviruses, JC or BK virus (BKV), are able to replicate in the kidney and/or cause systemic disease, and symptomatic infection with these agents can be associated with significant morbidity and mortality in immunocompromised host. While BK virus usually replicates in kidney transplant causing BK virus nephropathy (BKN) with characteristic decoy cells in the urine, CMV infection more often leads to systemic infection involving the gastrointestinal tract (GIT), lungs, or liver and can only sporadically be detected in renal transplant. In both cases, the disease is most often due to reactivation of a latent virus. Prevention and early treatment of posttransplant infection are therefore crucial with kidney transplant recipients. Since BKV viruria and viremia can be seen without renal injury and viral nephropathy, a diagnosis of BKN must be confirmed by renal biopsy. To date, preemptive treatment is the best strategy for CMV infection, while no available standard therapy, except for reduction of immunosuppression, is available for BKV infection.

Keywords: CMV, BK, cytomegalovirus, polyomavirus, viral infections, kidney transplantation

1. Introduction

CMV and polyomavirus infection is common in the human population and mainly remains asymptomatic through the life of healthy individuals. However, in immunocompromised individuals, such as kidney transplant recipients (KTRs), it can be associated with various complications, including direct systemic effects of viral infection, bacterial or fungal superinfection, viral infection of the transplanted kidney, and acute and chronic rejection, which consequently diminish patient and graft survival. Current preventive strategies in KTRs include preemptive therapy with valganciclovir or intravenous ganciclovir and universal prophylaxis with antivirals after kidney transplantation and for 1–3 months after treatment with antilymphocyte antibodies. Strategies to control established virus infection include decreasing immunosuppression, adding antivirals, and a combination of both [1–3].

BK virus nephropathy is the most common manifestation of BKV reactivation after renal transplantation, leading to loss of renal grafts in approximately 43% of patients. BKV viruria and viremia can be seen without renal injury and viral nephropathy, so renal biopsy remains the gold standard for definite BKN diagnosis. Therapeutic strategies of BKN management are still very limited, so screening protocols in order to detect early BK reactivation are important. BKN might be successfully managed with a reduction of baseline immunosuppression but is potentially harmful since it may be associated with increased risk of rejection [4–6].

2. CMV infection

CMV is a double-DNA virus of the herpesvirus family transmitted via saliva, body fluids, or tissue. There are various, species-specific strains of cytomegalovirus [7]. Seroprevalence ranges between 30 and 70% in Europe and North America. Following primary infection, CMV establishes latency in myeloid progenitor cells and can be transiently reactivated in a healthy host without causing disease, similar to polyomaviruses. However, CMV reactivates frequently and causes disease in KTRs in the setting of immunocompromised, typically in the first 2–3 months after transplantation [8, 9]. CMV viremia in the 1–6 months after transplantation is significantly more frequent in KTRs older than 65 years.

Reinfection (primary infection with a different human strain) can also occur [10].

CMV infection is the most common infectious disease following solid organ transplantation, including kidney [1, 3].

In addition to the direct effects of viral infection, CMV infection and disease have been associated with acute and chronic rejection and diminished patient and graft survival [2]. The transplanted kidney itself is only rarely affected by CMV reactivation.

The greatest recognized risk factor for CMV disease is a serological mismatch between the donor and the recipient (the recipient is CMV IgG seronegative and the donor is CMV IgG seropositive: D+/R−). Furthermore, CMV D+/R+ and CMV D−/R+ transplantations are of intermediate risk for the development of disease, and CMV D−/R− transplantation is considered as low risk (<5% incidence) [11, 12].

2.1 Definition

After the resolution of primary infection, CMV establishes latent infection. CMV can present in KTRs as either active CMV infection or CMV disease [9, 13].

Primary CMV infection: CMV infection in a person who was previously CMV seronegative (negative IgM and IgG CMV antibodies).

Latent CMV infection: after the resolution of acute (or primary) infection, CMV establishes latent infection. Patients who are CMV seropositive (IgG CMV antibodies) have latent infection. Secondary, symptomatic disease may present later, reflecting either reactivation of latent CMV or, less commonly, reinfection with a novel exogenous strain.

Active CMV infection is defined by CMV virus replication in plasma (viral load, viremia). CMV infection can be asymptomatic or symptomatic. The degree of immunosuppression in KTRs may determine progress to CMV disease.

CMV disease is defined as the presence of detectable CMV in a clinical specimen accompanied by other clinical manifestations. CMV disease may manifest as either CMV syndrome or tissue-invasive CMV disease [3].

2.2 Clinical features of CMV disease

2.2.1 CMV syndrome

For a determination of CMV syndrome, CMV in plasma (quantitative PCR CMV DNA (PCR)) and the presence of at least one of the following symptoms and signs of disease are necessary: fever ≥38°C, general signs (malaise, myalgia, arthralgias), leukopenia (≤3.5 × 10^9/L), atypical lymphocytosis (≥5%), and thrombocytopenia (≤100 × 10^9/L). In a case of suspected CMV nephritis in KTRs, kidney graft rejection should always be ruled out [3].

2.2.2 Tissue-invasive disease

In a case of tissue-invasive CMV disease, evidence of particular tissue/organ involvement (hepatitis, colitis, pancreatitis, pneumonitis, nephritis, cystitis, etc.) is based on clinical symptoms and signs associated with a particular organ, positive quantitative PCR CMV DNA in plasma, and, in particular, on the presence of CMV in a given organ or tissue (detected by methods of isolation, histopathology, immunohistochemistry, or hybridization in situ). CMV invasive disease can be most frequently detected in the intestine (40%) followed by the liver (20%), lungs (10%), kidneys (5%), and eyes/brain (1%) [8]. For CMV encephalitis, it is sufficient to prove the presence of CMV in the liquor (PCR) and for CMV pneumonitis in bronchoalveolar flushing (PCR).

In suspected CMV retinitis, ophthalmological examination is sufficient for the diagnosis. In patients with tissue-invasive disease (particularly in CMV infection of the central nervous system, chorioretinitis, and in CMV infection of the gut), CMV viremia may be absent, so some more invasive diagnostics (lumbar puncture, sigmoidoscopy/colonoscopy) must be proceeded in case of clinical suspicion [14].

2.3 Diagnosis

In KTRs who present with signs and symptoms suspicious for CMV disease, laboratory confirmation is required to establish the diagnosis. A biopsy with histopathologic examination of tissue is occasionally necessary to diagnose tissue-invasive CMV disease.

A diagnosis of CMV infection is most often confirmed with nucleic acid testing using polymerase chain reaction (PCR) for the detection of CMV DNA. PCR is primarily used to evaluate blood, cerebrospinal fluid, and ocular or vitreous fluid, although various clinical specimens can be subjected to this assay.

Among other tests to detect CMV, the demonstration of CMV p65 antigen in circulating polymorphonuclear leukocytes in the buffy coat has been used both to monitor response to therapy and as a guide to starting treatment in some centers. Traditional viral cultures are rarely used to diagnose CMV [15].

The most common serologic tests that detect CMV antibodies (IgM and IgG antibody to CMV) are based on enzyme-linked immunosorbent assay (ELISA). A positive test for CMV IgG indicates that a person was infected with CMV at some time during their life. The presence of CMV IgM cannot be used by itself to diagnose primary CMV infection because IgM can persist for months after primary infection and because IgM can be positive in reactivated CMV infections [16].

On occasion histopathological confirmation of CMV disease is necessary to prove CMV organ-specific dysfunction.

2.4 Histological features of tissue-invasive disease

Productive CMV infection in the tissue is characterized by a cytopathic viral effect in the biopsy specimen of parenchymal organs and the presence of CMV-positive cells by immunohistochemistry or by in situ hybridization with antibody directed against the immediate early antigen. Additionally, CMV virions may be detected by electron microscopy [17].

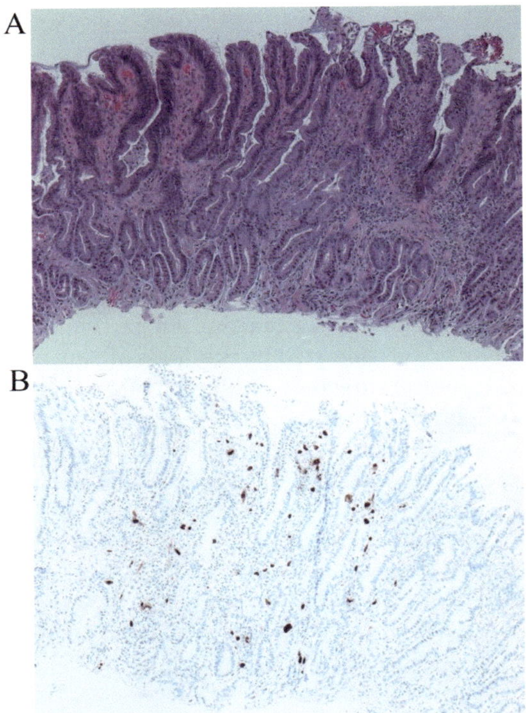

Figure 1.
CMV gastritis with focal active and chronic inflammation (A, Trichrome stain, 100x). Immunohistochemical stain against CMV antigen shows numerous CMV-positive cells (B, CMV, 100x).

In daily practice, CMV reactivation is most frequently detected in GIT biopsies, including the colon and stomach (**Figure 1**). In contrast to polyomaviruses, CMV invasive disease is only sporadically detected in transplanted kidney [18, 19]. Histological features of CMV replication-related lesions in native kidneys are similar to those in renal transplants [20, 21].

2.4.1 CMV disease in kidneys

CMV nephritis is characterized by virally induced direct tissue injury and by biopsy-proven cytopathic changes. Cytopathic changes are typically focal and detected in tubular epithelial cells or endothelial cells (**Figure 2**).

Three patterns have been observed: pattern I with large intranuclear inclusions in tubular epithelial cells with interstitial nephritis, pattern II with central large eosinophilic intranuclear inclusions in endothelial cells, and rarely, CMV infection may occur as acute glomerulonephritis (pattern III) [18]. CMV infection may also affect podocytes.

In the predominant tubular involvement, tubular CMV infection is usually accompanied by variable interstitial inflammation. In addition, monocyte inclusions in the interstitial infiltrate may be observed. Occasionally, a dense nodular mononuclear and plasma cell infiltrate is present in the interstitium, sometimes reminiscent of granuloma. Focal necrosis and microabscesses are rarely observed. Prominent tubulitis reminiscent of T-cell-mediated rejection characteristic in BKN is absent.

The involvement of endothelial cells is characterized by a central large eosinophilic intranuclear inclusions surrounded by a circumferential halo resembling a typical owl's eye. Glomerular and peritubular capillary endothelial cells may

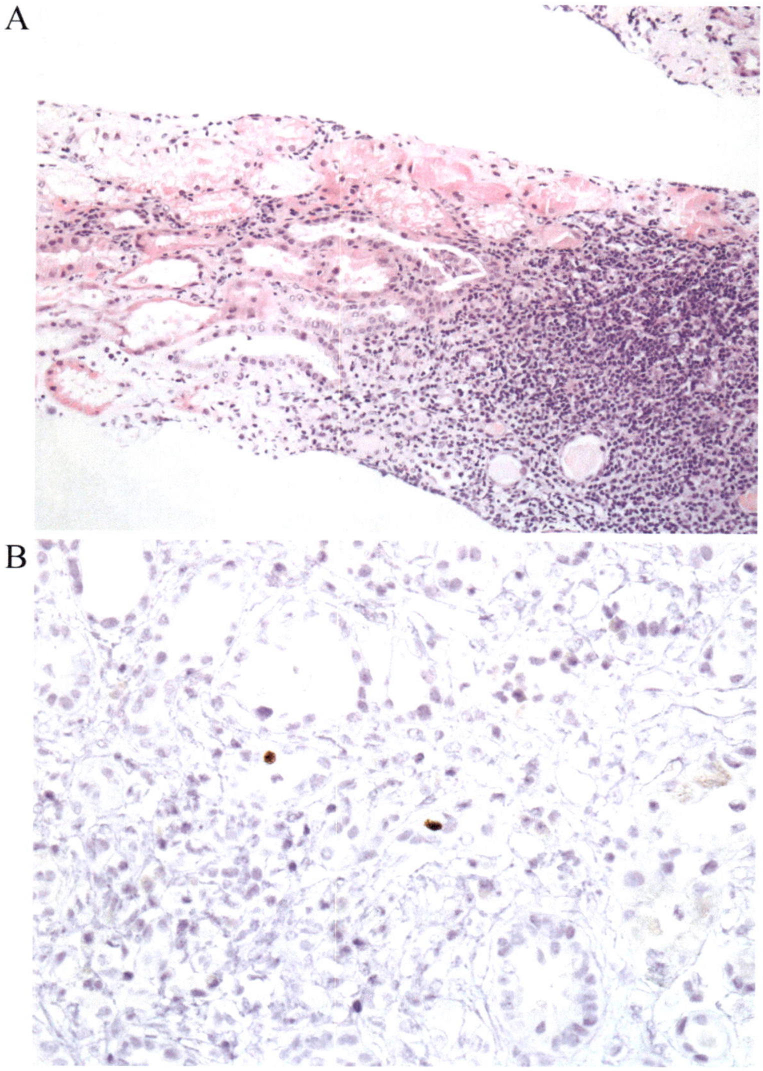

Figure 2.
CMV nephritis in transplanted kidney: focal interstitial inflammation and cytopathic changes in scarce tubular epithelial cells (A, hematoxylin eosin (HE), 200x). CMV inclusions are confirmed by immunohistochemistry (B, CMV, 400x). Courtesy of Danica Galešič Ljubanović and Petar Šenjug.

be infected. In some nuclei, a smudgy-appearing intranuclear inclusion can be detected. In the cytoplasm of viral-infected cells, there are sometimes small basophilic cytoplasmic viral inclusions. When endothelial cells are predominantly CMV-infected cells, tubular epithelium tends to be spared. In such cases, interstitial inflammation is not prominent [18].

Immunofluorescence with a standard panel of antibodies is usually unremarkable, only rarely are scarce glomerular IgG deposits detected [20–22].

CMV nephritis may be associated with concurrent antibody- and T-cell-mediated rejection in 30% of cases [22]. In contrast to polyomavirus, CMV often replicates in endothelial and inflammatory cells. Distinction between infection-driven inflammation and rejection may be difficult.

Immunomodulation of the immune response might be the most important indirect effect of CMV infection on kidney graft, rather than direct CMV nephritis.

It is considered to promote rejection episodes by stimulating a T-cell-mediated response. Reinke reported that 85% of patients with late-acute renal allograft rejection with otherwise symptomless CMV infection responded to ganciclovir therapy, which emphasized the indirect role of CMV infection on graft function [23]. CMV infection does not activate classic complement pathway nor trigger the deposition of complement factor C4d along peritubular capillaries; in the case of positive C4d deposition, concurrent ABMR should be considered.

2.4.2 CMV disease in gastrointestinal tract

Cytomegalovirus infection of the gastrointestinal tract is the most common manifestation of tissue-invasive CMV disease and is a significant cause of morbidity and mortality in the solid organ transplantation recipients. Patients usually present with esophagitis, colitis, and hepatitis; however, infection can occur anywhere in the gastrointestinal tract [17, 24, 25].

Mucosal ulceration was the most common endoscopic finding present in 75% of cases (**Figure 3**). Other endoscopic features include mucosal edema, hyperemia, and nodularity. In a renal transplant patient, cytomegalovirus infection may rarely present as a localized disease, such as inflammatory polyps [26].

Two histologic patterns of GIT tissue injury have been described. In the first form, viral inclusions are typically found in the glandular epithelium with little associated tissue reaction (**Figure 4**). In the second form, CMV inclusions are found in swollen endothelial and stromal cells, especially in areas of ulceration. Typically, mucosal erosion, ulceration, hemorrhage, necrosis, perforation, and/or fistula formation can be detected. CMV colitis is characterized by uneven inflammation in the lamina propria, with active changes and ulcers with abundant purulent exudate (**Figures 3** and **5**) [24].

In contrast to other organs, CMV infection in the colon does not always produce the diagnostic large cells with viral inclusions with owl's eye appearance. Rather, the infected cells can be smaller, up to twice as big as their normal counterparts, and have small basophilic inclusions, often with no characteristic clear halo. They have been called "atypical inclusions" [27].

Diagnosis is usually by histopathology with immunohistochemistry or viral culture of tissue specimens; molecular assays such as quantitative PCR also often have a role (**Figures 4** and **5**).

However, there is little consensus on the specificity of PCR [28–30]. Since CMV typically produces latent infection residing in leukocytes, concern has been raised that positive PCR might therefore not necessarily reflect active disease in the colon but only latent infection. The use of colon tissue alone was therefore not widely considered to provide definitive proof of CMV colitis [13]. Zidar et al. observed good correlation among the density of positive cells by immunohistochemistry, the

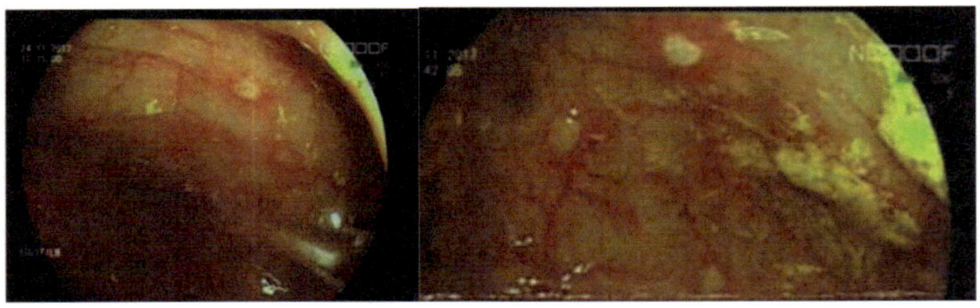

Figure 3.
Mucosal ulcerations in CMV colitis of kidney transplant recipient are common endoscopic findings.

DOI: http://dx.doi.org/10.5772/intechopen.86043

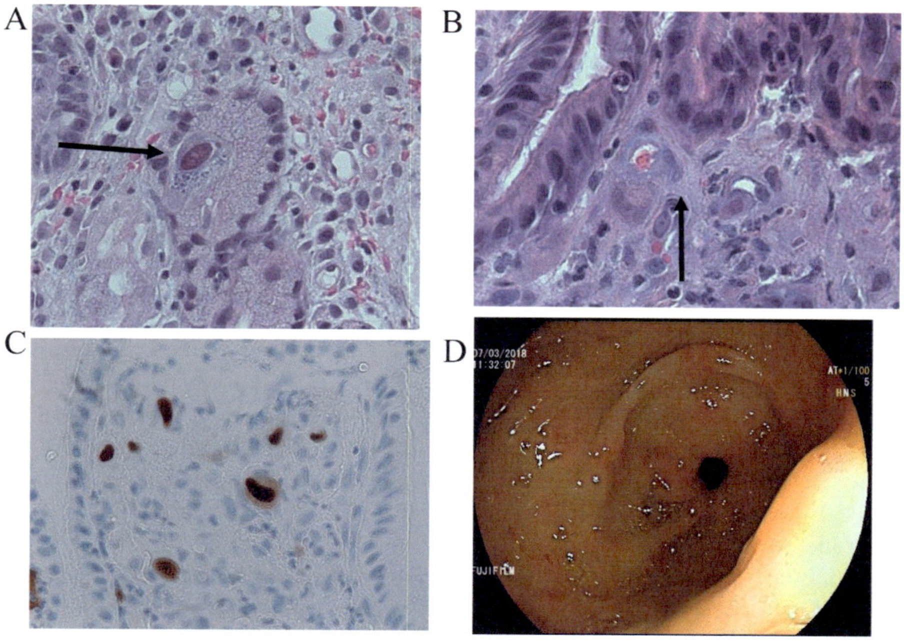

Figure 4.
CMV gastritis. Intranuclear inclusion (arrow) in foveolar gastric cell (A) and in endothelial cell (arrow) of a capillary in the lamina propria (both Thricrome stain, 600x). CMV positive Intranuclear inclusions by immunohistochemistry (C, CMV, 600x). Scarce mucosal ulcerations seen on gastroscopy (D).

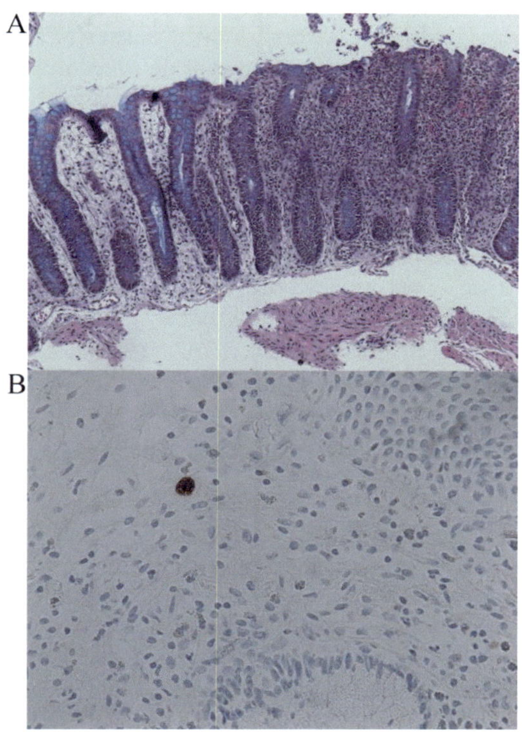

Figure 5.
CMV colitis in kidney transplant recipient. Focal active colitis with erosions (A, Trichrome stain, 100x). There was only one positive CMV cell by immunohistochemistry (CMV, 400x).

morphology, and the number of viral copies by qPCR in IBD patients. Both immunohistochemistry and qPCR can therefore be successfully used for diagnosing CMV reactivation, at least in CMV reactivation in patients with IBD. The optimal sites for endoscopic biopsies to obtain specimens with the highest values of CMV are the base and the edge of ulcers [28, 31].

2.5 Prevention of CMV disease

CMV can be prevented in two ways: by prophylaxis and by preemptive treatment. Both options are effective for preventing CMV disease [32–34].

2.5.1 CMV prophylaxis therapy

CMV prophylaxis is widely used in the transplantation setting and has been associated with reductions in CMV disease, mortality, and graft rejection. Prophylaxis refers to the administration of antiviral drugs to all patients (universal prophylaxis) or to a subgroup of patients at higher risk of viral replication (specific prophylaxis) for a predetermined period of time. In KTRs, prophylaxis therapy aims to prevent CMV infection and, consequently, CMV-associated disease. According to current guidelines, universal prophylaxis is recommended in patients with high risk (i.e., those who have D+/R− CMV IgG or who have received T-cell depletion for induction prior to transplantation). Antiviral drug treatment should begin immediately after transplantation or after the use of antilymphocyte antibodies. Patients with low to intermediate risk can undergo preemptive treatment instead of prophylaxis [35].

Until recently, the emphasis on prophylaxis with prophylactic agents focused on early disease occurring in high-risk patients, with the duration of prophylaxis typically no longer than 3 months. Although early-onset CMV infection was usually sufficiently controlled, the reported incidence of delayed-onset CMV infection following the completion of a 3-month course of preventive therapy was high, and, consequently, prophylactic therapy in most centers was extended to 6 months in the group of KTRs at most risk (D+/R−) [36, 37].

Several medications are available: acyclovir, valacyclovir, intravenous ganciclovir, oral ganciclovir, and valganciclovir. Ganciclovir takes precedence over acyclovir. In a clinical setting, the most commonly used medication for prophylaxis is oral valganciclovir with dose adjustment according to kidney function [38].

The prophylaxis should be initiated immediately after transplantation. The decision on the duration of prophylaxis depends on the CMV serostatus of the donor (D) and recipient (R), of the organ transplant, and the degree of immune deficiency in the transplant recipient.

2.5.1.1 Prophylaxis in D+/R− recipient

In D+/R−, prophylaxis should last for 3–6 months. According to recent research, many transplant centers are opting for a 6-month prophylaxis, which has been associated with a significant decrease in the incidence of late CMV disease, compared to 3-month prophylaxis. Valganciclovir at a dosage of 900 mg orally once daily with the dose adjusted for renal function is used in most centers for a period of 6 months following transplantation.

2.5.1.2 Prophylaxis in D+/R+ or D−/R+

In D+/R+ or D−/R+, prophylaxis should last for 3 months. Extension to 6 months is suggested for KTRs who have received antilymphocyte antibody induction. Valganciclovir at 900 mg orally once daily for 3 months following transplantation, with the dose adjusted for renal function, is the standard prophylactic therapy in most centers.

2.5.1.3 Prophylaxis in D−/R−

There is little risk of CMV infection in these patients. Precautions for transfusion of blood and blood products of CMV-positive donors are required [35].

2.5.2 Additional considerations in the prevention of CMV in kidney transplant recipients

2.5.2.1 CMV matching

Theoretically, a method of minimizing the risk of CMV infection would be to avoid transplantation of a seropositive organ into a seronegative recipient. Historically, before the advent of antiviral prophylaxis, many units avoided transplanting CMV-positive solid organs into CMV-negative recipients. However, given the shortage of donor organs, such an approach is difficult to practice in these settings.

One area in which CMV matching remains relevant is in the elective use of blood products. Where it is known that both donor and recipient are seronegative for CMV, leukodepleted blood and blood products are available and should be used to minimize the risk of primary infection [39].

2.5.2.2 Passive immunoprophylaxis

Passive immunoprophylaxis has been explored in solid organ transplantation in a number of randomized trials, whereby hyperimmune globulin provided significant overall protection from severe disease, with a reduced rate of CMV disease to approximately half of that seen in the placebo groups. Intravenous treatment is generally less convenient for the patient and health-care provider and carries the theoretical risk of transmitting blood-borne viruses [39].

2.5.3 Preemptive therapy

With quantitative monitoring of CMV DNA in plasma (viral load, viremia) once a week (sometimes twice a week), CMV viremia can be detected before the occurrence of symptomatic infection. However, the exact cutoff point of plasma CMV concentration to initiate preemptive treatment (from a few hundred to several thousand copies of CMV DNA in 1 ml of plasma) is not known. The decision to initiate preemptive treatment is therefore individual and depends mainly on the degree and duration of immunosuppression [40].

The benefits of this type of strategy are that fewer patients are exposed to antivirals and for a shorter period of time (fewer side effects, fewer interactions with other medicines, lower costs).

Intravenous ganciclovir (5 mg/kg every 12 h or a dose adjusted to creatinine clearance) is used for preemptive treatment in a patient with a high viral load (>50,000 copies of CMV DNA in 1 ml of plasma), in severe renal impairment, and in pediatric patients; otherwise, valganciclovir (900 mg every 12 h, or a dose adjusted to creatinine clearance) is recommended. If there is no CMV disease, the CMV viremia is checked for the first time after 7–10 days of preemptive treatment, afterward being monitored every 7–10 days. It is recommended to continue with preemptive therapy until two negative results of quantitative plasma PCR CMV DNA tests performed in a space of 7 days [40].

2.5.3.1 Guiding of preemptive therapy by measurement of CMV-specific T lymphocytes

The activity and concentration of CMV-specific lymphocytes in the blood have a decisive role in controlling CMV infection, especially in situations of increased risk of CMV reactivation or primary infection, such as after therapeutic use of antilymphocyte antibodies. The count of CMV-specific T lymphocytes allows a decision on preemptive treatment in a period when the viral load is still not critically increased.

Among the available methods, the most reliable predictor of viremia and disease is measurement of the blood concentration of T lymphocytes, which, after in vitro stimulation with CMV peptides, increasingly produce cytokines such as interferon gamma and interleukin 2. CMV-specific lymphocytes CD4 and CD8 are analyzed by the flow cytometry method (one of the most commonly used is a whole blood interferon gamma release assay QuantiFERON-CMV test marketed by an Australian company, Cellestis Inc., which measures the production of interferon gamma after stimulating the patient's lymphocytes with CMV peptides) [41].

2.6 Treatment of CMV disease

Treatment is always indicated in case of active CMV infection (CMV viral syndrome) or in the presence of tissue-invasive CMV disease [42].

Intravenous ganciclovir is a gold standard for the treatment of CMV disease. In mild to moderate cases of the disease, oral valganciclovir was found to be non-inferior to intravenous ganciclovir. However, due to limited evidence, severe disease should be treated with intravenous ganciclovir. Acyclovir and valacyclovir are not indicated for treatment. The use of foscarnet as a first-line therapy is limited by its toxicity (mainly nephrotoxicity) (**Table 1**).

Drug resistance should be suspected in patients with persistent viral replication and/or clinical progression after 2–3 weeks of treatment. Ganciclovir-resistant CMV infection has been observed in 1–2% of kidney transplant recipients and is a result of the widespread use of antiviral prophylaxis and preemptive therapy. Drug resistance typically develops in CMV D+/R− patients and is also associated with high viral load, prolonged antiviral therapy, high level of immunosuppression (i.e., use of antilymphocyte antibodies), and suboptimal serum drug concentrations. Genotypic tests reveal characteristic viral mutants (UL97) associated with resistance [43].

Drug-resistant or refractory CMV disease occasionally responds to an increased dose of ganciclovir. In cases of genotypic resistance of CMV to ganciclovir, it is necessary to introduce combined treatment with ganciclovir and foscarnet (half or standard doses) or treat with foscarnet only [44].

The treatment should be continuous until viral eradication is achieved in two assays after a minimum of 2 weeks of induction treatment. Initial treatment with intravenous ganciclovir can be later replaced with oral valganciclovir. During the course of treatment, renal function must be promptly monitored. In most cases (especially in high viremia, a moderate to severe clinical course, ganciclovir resistance), it is necessary to reduce immunosuppressive therapy (especially antimetabolites, i.e., azathioprine or mycophenolate). The same applies in cases of recurrent CMV infection/disease [35].

In the case of high-risk patients, some authors recommend secondary prophylaxis after completion of treatment, although no consensus has so far been achieved on this approach [35, 45].

DOI: http://dx.doi.org/10.5772/intechopen.86043

Drug	Dosage	Action	Formulation	Common side effects
Ganciclovir	5 mg/kg bw i.v.; adjusted to eGF * Oral preparation has low bioavailability	Competitive inhibition of DNA synthesis catalyzed by the viral DNA polymerase	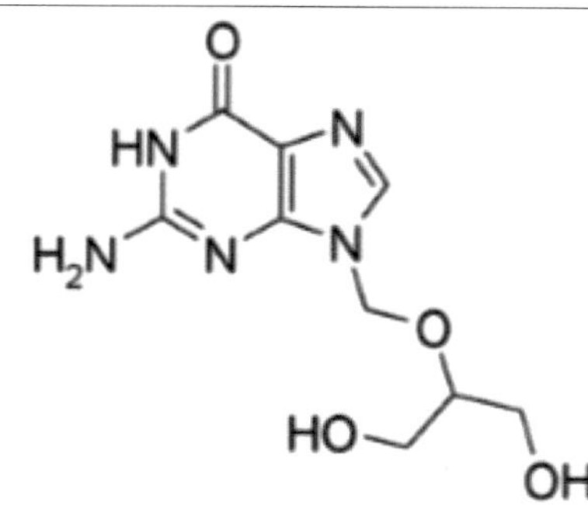	Leukopenia, thrombocytopenia, diarrhea, long-term reproductive toxicity
Valganciclovir	900 mg bd p.o.; adjusted to eGF	Rapidly metabolized into active form (ganciclovir) in the intestinal wall and liver; same action as ganciclovir	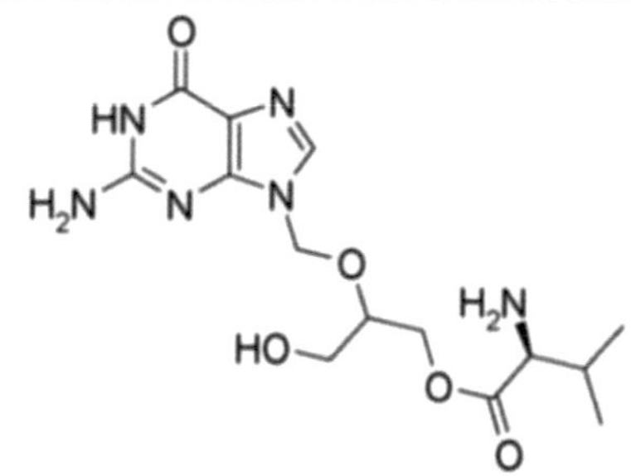	Leukopenia, thrombocytopenia, anemia, gastrointestinal toxicity
Foscarnet	90 mg/kg bw bd i.v. or 60 mg/kg bw every 8 h; adjusted to eGF	Inhibits activity to the viral DNA polymerase by binding to the pyrophosphate binding site and blocking cleavage of pyrophosphate from the terminal nucleoside triphosphate added to the growing DNA chain	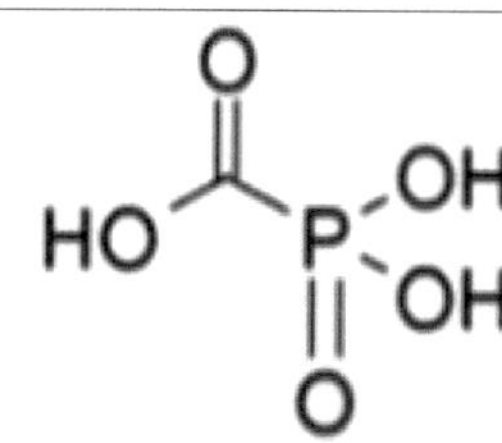	Nephrotoxicity, electrolyte disturbances, neurotoxicity

Drug	Dosage	Action	Formulation	Common side effects
Cidofovir	5 mg/kg i.v. once a week for 2 consecutive weeks. Following induction dose, 5 mg/kg i.v. once every 2 weeks administer with probenecid to decrease side effects to the kidney	After conversion to active form, cidofovir diphosphate competitively inhibits DNA polymerase	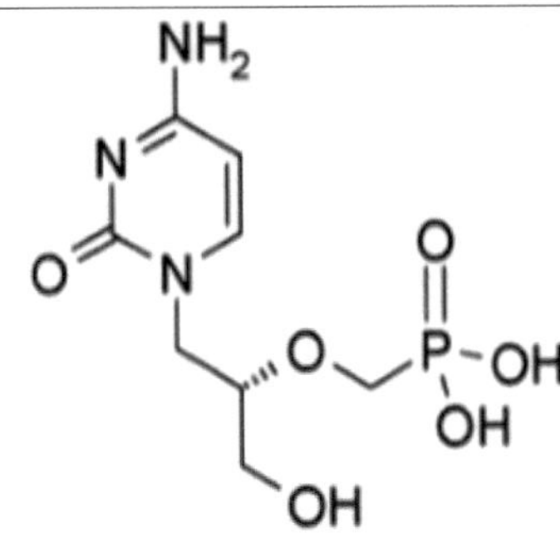	Nephrotoxicity, neutropenia, teratogenicity, carcinogenicity, nausea, vomiting
Maribavir	To be determined	Inhibits UL97 kinase and stops viral maturation and egress	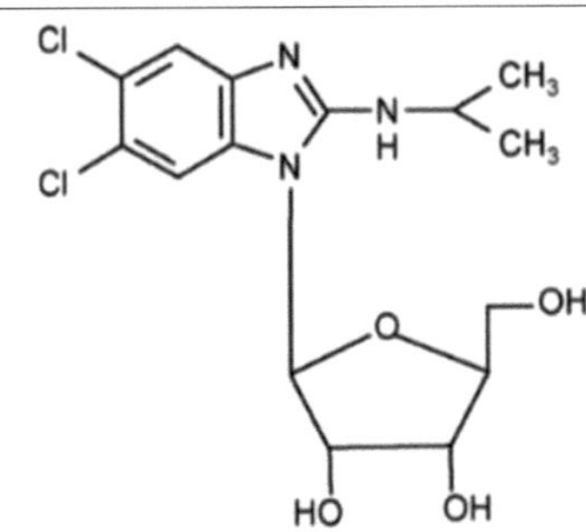	Taste disturbance; inferior at preventing CMV disease

i.v., intravenous; p.o., peroral; eGF, estimated glomerular filtration.

Table 1.
Drugs used in therapy of CMV disease.

3. BK polyomavirus infection and disease in humans

Polyomaviruses are non-enveloped, double-stranded ubiquitous DNA viruses living in birds and mammals as natural hosts. The name indicates their ability to produce tumors (Greek poly- many, multiple; -oma, tumors), particularly in rodents and experimental models [46].

Seroprevalence in humans ranges from 20 to 90%, depending on the viral strain and patient age. It generally remains asymptomatic in the renourinary tract of healthy individuals, although may undergo periods of self-limiting transient asymptomatic activation with viruria and viremia, without causing disease [46]. However, in immunocompromised individuals, such as renal transplant recipients, it can be associated with various patterns of tissue injury, of which BK virus nephropathy is the most common.

Among approximately 18 polyomavirus strains, BK virus, JC virus, and simian virus (SV-40) have been considered to be pathogenic in humans. Infections with SV-40 were detected following the administration of contaminated polio vaccines in the late 1950s, without known clinical manifestation in humans [46].

BK virus was isolated in 1971 from a patient with ureteral stenosis after kidney transplantation and was named after the initials of the infected patient. Similarly, JC virus was named after a patient with progressive multifocal leukoencephalopathy. Both strains are characterized by productive viral infection with tissue injury, showing specific tropism for the renourinary tract or central nervous system [46, 47].

Recent studies have indicated that BK virus may be involved in the tumorigenesis of bladder carcinoma in renal transplant recipients and salivary gland inflammation and sclerosis in HIV patients [48, 49]. Trichodysplasia spinulosa-associated polyomavirus and Merkel cell carcinoma polyomavirus, recently detected new strains, may be related to proliferative lesions and neoplasms without productive viral replication [50].

3.1 BK nephropathy

PVN is a major causative agent in nephropathy after renal transplantation, affecting 1–10% of patients [51].

In the past, when immunosuppressive therapy was based mainly on cyclosporine, only sporadic PVN cases were reported. Although modern immunosuppressive drugs introduced after 1990 have enabled less rejection and improved allograft survival, they have been responsible for the occurrence of previously uncommon side effects, including PVN and hemorrhagic cystitis [47].

Before screening protocols for PV reactivation in renal transplant recipients were routinely used, PVN was usually diagnosed late after transplantation, in an advanced histologic stage, with chronic renal changes leading to allograft loss within 1 year in 50–90% of cases [4, 50]. Potential misdiagnosis of concurrent rejection resulting in increased immunosuppression might contribute to accelerated allograft failure.

3.2 Features of BKN

PVN is typically caused by the BK strain and only rarely by simultaneous activation of BK and JC viruses. The specific viral activation mechanisms remain unknown [47]. The transplant microenvironment may promote viral reactivation, because only sporadic detection of PV in native kidney of patients with other organ transplants or in immunodeficient patients has been reported [52, 53]. PVN also commonly occurs in patients with posttransplantation complications, including

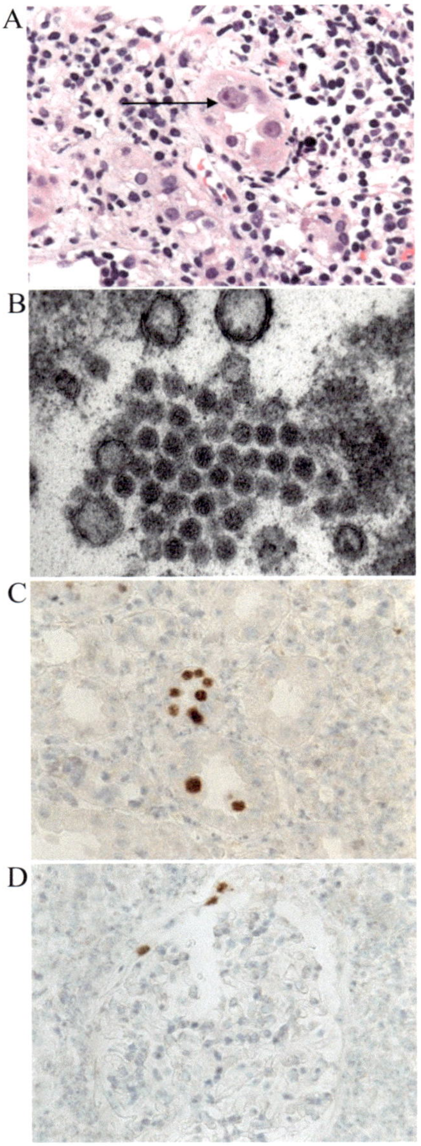

Figure 6.
Diagnosis of BK nephropathy: intranuclear viral inclusion bodies in tubular epithelial cells (A, HE, 200x), intracellular virions of 40–50 nm in diameter by electron microscopy (B, electron micrograph), intranuclear expression of SV-40 antigen in tubular epithelial cells (C) and/or epithelial cells of Bowman's capsule (D, both SV-40, 400x).

delayed graft function and acute rejection. Other risk factors are male gender, older recipient age, diabetes, prolonged ureteral stent placement, smoldering subclinical graft inflammation, and/or abnormalities of dendritic cell and NK cell/T-cell activation. Relative over-immunosuppression by modern immunosuppressive drugs, though, is considered the main risk factor [47, 51, 54].

Polyomavirus infection represents serological or virological evidence of virus exposure without distinguishing among replicating, latent, and transforming patterns. Manifest viral disease is, however, defined as histological evidence of polyomavirus-mediated organ pathology and is mainly limited to immunocompromised patients, such as transplant recipients [47, 55, 56].

Recognition of BKN is critical, since the proper therapy is reduction, rather than enhanced immunosuppression.

3.3 Diagnosis of BKN

In order to confirm intrarenal BKV replication, renal biopsy remains the gold standard for a definitive diagnosis of BKN [51]. A minimum of two cores including the medulla are recommended to make a correct diagnosis, since in the early stage, viral inclusions may be present only in the medulla [5, 51, 57]. However, characteristic viral inclusion and tubular injury might be focally observed in the biopsy specimens, so PVN can be missed due to sampling error (**Figure 6**).

3.3.1 Morphological characteristics of BKN

BKN is morphologically characterized by intrarenal viral replication, mainly in tubular epithelial cell nuclei (intranuclear inclusions), causing tubular injury, shedding of tubular epithelial cells, and cell lysis (**Figures 7** and **8**). On immunofluorescence, focal immune complex-type granular deposition of IG along the tubular basement membrane is sometimes found, indicating BK infection (**Figure 9**), although the biologic and clinical significance of this finding needs further evaluation [5].

Viral replication in tubular epithelial cells can induce various nuclear changes: an amorphous ground-glass inclusion body (type 1), a central irregular inclusion body surrounded by a halo (type 2), finely granular nuclear alterations (type 3), and vesicular changes with coarsely clumped viral inclusions (type 4) (**Figure 10**).

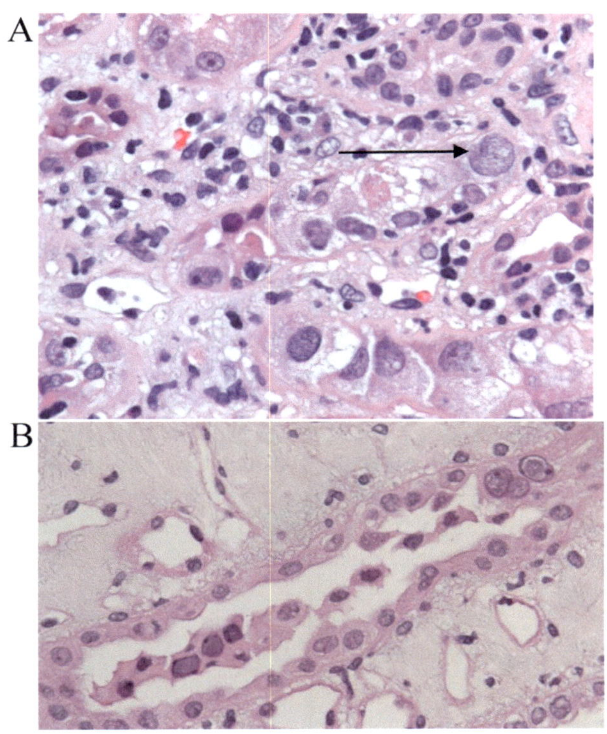

Figure 7.
BK virus nephropathy. Virally induced tubular epithelial cell injury and lysis in cortex (A, HE, 200x) and medulla (B, HE, 100x). Intranuclear viral inclusion bodies are observed (arrow).

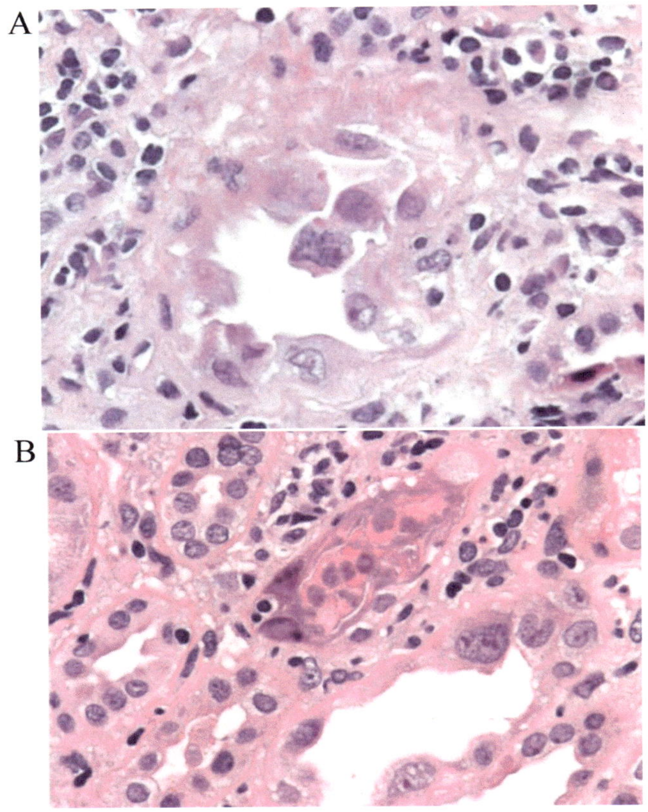

Figure 8.
Virally induced tubular epithelial cells with intranuclear inclusions, shedding of infected cells, tubular injury, and lysis (A,HE, 400x and B, HE, 200x).

In rare cases, the ascending PV infection can affect the parietal epithelial cells of Bowman's capsule, mainly detected by immunohistochemistry (**Figure 6**).

Diagnostic confirmation can easily be achieved by immunohistochemistry (**Figure 6**) or immunofluorescence, with antibodies directed against the polyomavirus T antigen, VP capsid proteins, or detection of intracellular virions of 40–50 nm in diameter by electron microscopy (**Figure 11**) [5, 57].

In early stages of PVN with focal and minimal tubular changes without tubular injury and characteristic intranuclear inclusions, a diagnosis can only be established by immunohistochemistry with antibody directed against SV-40-T antigen (**Figure 12**). Later in the course of the disease, many cases of PVN may show numerous infected cells and an inflammatory lymphocytic infiltrate with tubulitis mimicking acute T-cell-mediated rejection (**Figure 13**). Advanced disease, detected late after transplantation, often shows marked interstitial fibrosis/tubular atrophy, while interstitial inflammation and viral replication may be variable (**Figure 14**).

3.4 Differential diagnosis of BKN

PVN must be differentiated from other rare viral infections, including CMV, herpes simplex virus, and adenovirus. CMV disease in transplant recipients is more frequent than BKN and usually affects the intestine, liver, or lungs but only rarely manifests as CMV reactivation in renal graft. Since the histological features of BKN

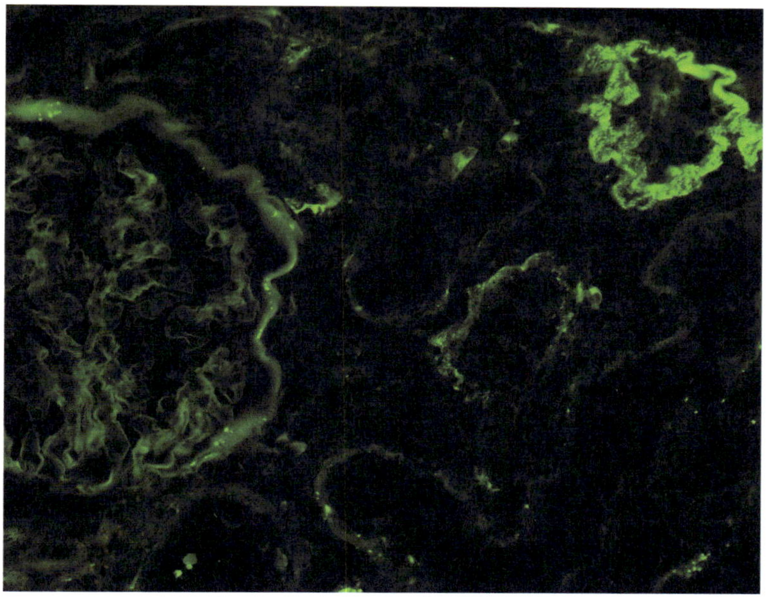

Figure 9.
On immunofluorescence, focal immune complex-type granular deposition of IgG along the tubular basement membrane is sometimes found.

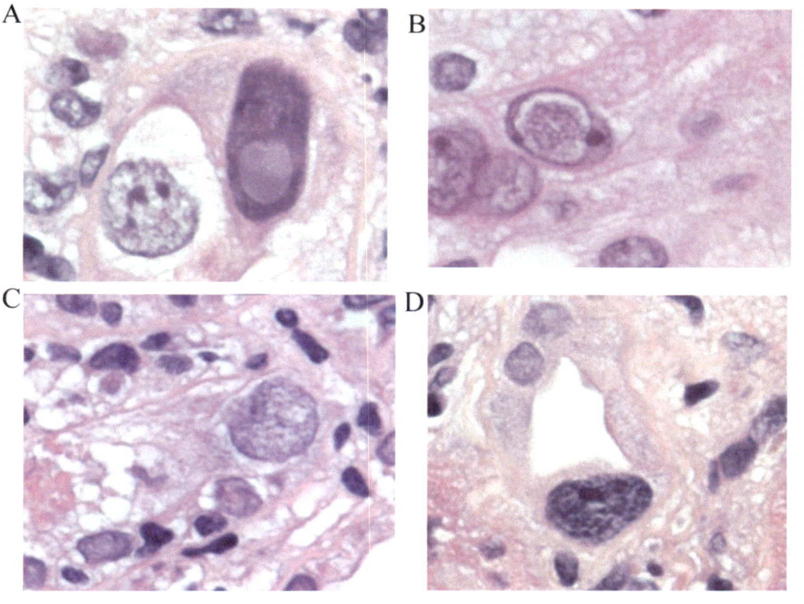

Figure 10.
Various nuclear changes induced by viral replication: type 1, an amorphous ground-glass inclusion body (A); type 2, a central irregular inclusion body surrounded by nuclear halo (B); type 3, finely granular nuclear alteration (C); type 4, vesicular nuclear changes with coarsely clumped viral inclusions (D, all HE, 600x).

may overlap with other viral infections, specific immunohistochemical staining is a sensitive tool for differentiating among BK, CMV, adenovirus, or herpes simplex viral infection. The main histological features of common transplant kidney viral infection are shown in **Table 2**.

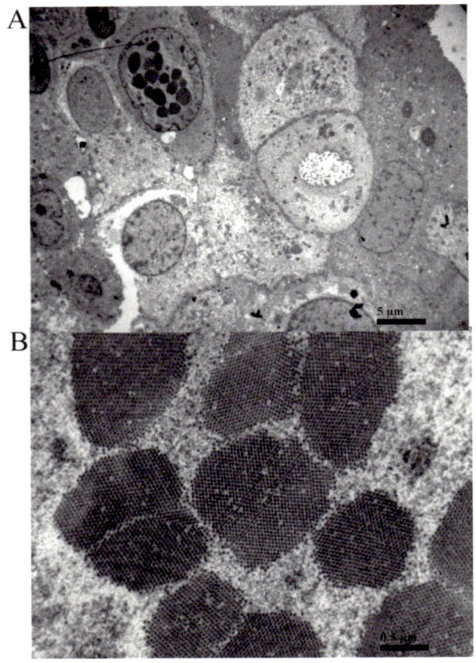

Figure 11.
Intranuclear viral inclusions in a tubular epithelial cell (A). Intranuclear virions measuring 40–50 nm in diameter (B, electron micrographs).

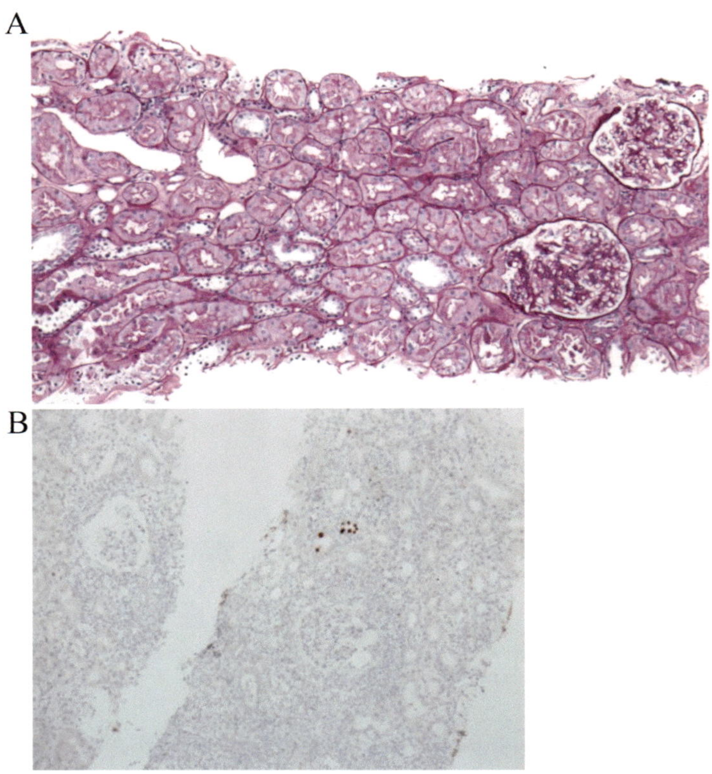

Figure 12.
BKN grade 1. Early phase with only focal tubular injury. (A, HE, 100x) and few SV-40 positive cells on immunohistochemistry (B, SV-40, 100x).

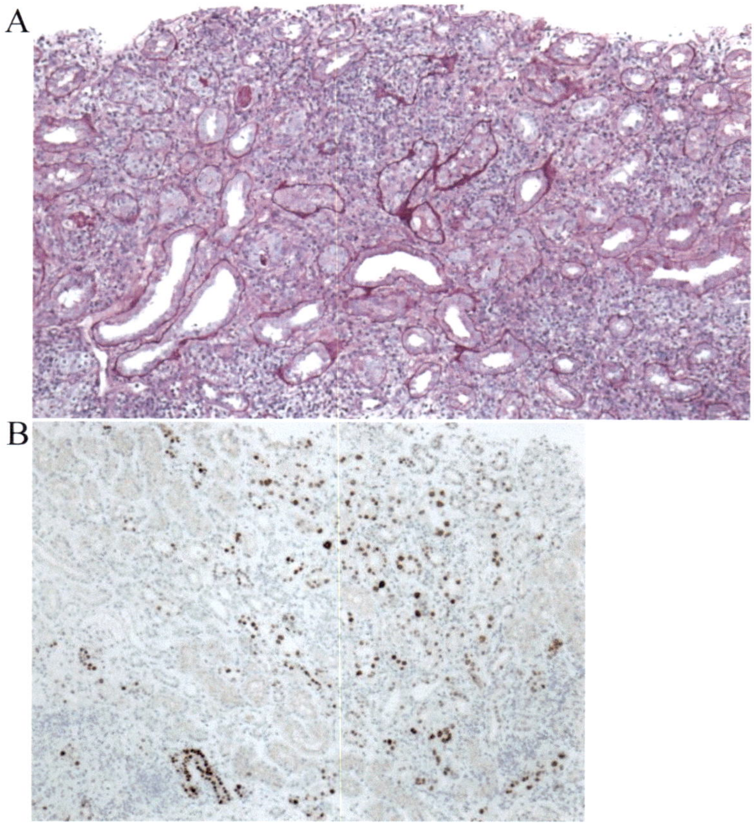

Figure 13.
BKN grade 2. Florid phase with severe interstitial inflammation and tubulitis in BK nephropathy, indistinguishable from acute rejection. There was no endarteritis (A, PAS, 200x). Numerous BK-positive cells on immunohistochemistry were detected. (SV-40, 200×).

However, the most important differential diagnosis, particularly in PVN after reduction of immunosuppression, remains T-cell-mediated acute rejection [6]. Careful correlations with clinical data, such as the presence of donor-specific antibodies, recent immunosuppression reduction, DNA viral load in the serum, and presence of decoy cells in the urine, provide additional information in order to make a correct diagnosis. Glomeruli and vessels must be carefully examined in order to exclude glomerulitis and vasculitis, which would strongly suggest concomitant rejection. C4d positivity and diffuse peritubular capillaritis outside the area of extensive interstitial inflammation, together with positive donor-specific antibodies (DSA), are consistent with concomitant antibody-mediated rejection.

A diagnosis of PVN and concomitant T-cell-mediated rejection after immunosuppression reduction is challenging and needs careful correlation of biopsy findings with the dynamics of BK viremia. Focal interstitial inflammation in the context of stable graft function and recently cleared BK viremia should be interpreted as residual BKN, but the same histology findings detected beyond 3 months after BK clearance, accompanied by a rise in serum creatinine, might rather point toward acute rejection.

3.5 Course of BKN

The natural course of BKN remains to be elucidated. Some authors have reported that biopsies obtained after reduction of immunosuppression during

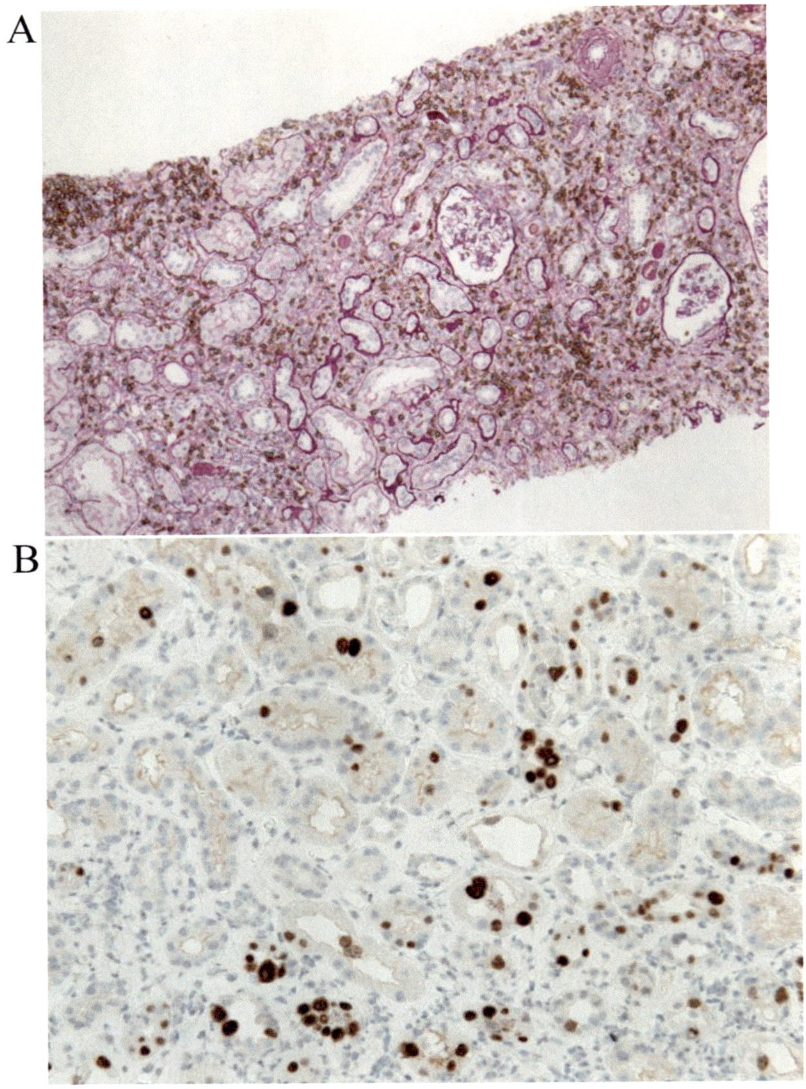

Figure 14.
BKN grade 3. Moderate interstitial fibrosis/tubular atrophy and interstitial inflammation composed of CD3 positive lymphocytes in areas of fibrosis (A, CD3 and PAS, 100x). Many tubules show viral replication (B, SV-40 antigen, 200x).

decrease of the plasma viral load may show severe interstitial infiltrate and tubulitis reminiscent of T-cell-mediated acute rejection, but the outcome of renal grafts was good despite prolonged reduction of immunosuppression without corticosteroid administration [4, 6, 58, 59]. Such patients typically presented with a transient increase in serum creatinine, accompanied by a decrease in plasma viral load, which finally disappeared [59]. Moreover, serum creatinine returned to the baseline level after a few months. In subsequent biopsies, the virus was cleared from renal tissue, and inflammation resolved without the presence of marked interstitial fibrosis. These authors have suggested that such tubulointerstitial nephritis might be immune reconstitution-associated graft inflammation, enabling the resolution of PVN.

	Polyomavirus	Cytomegalovirus
Viral inclusions	Type 1: an amorphous ground-glass inclusion body Type 2: a central irregular inclusion body surrounded by nuclear halo Type 3: finely granular nuclear alteration Type 4: finely granular nuclear alteration	Smudgy/ground-glass nuclear inclusions surrounded by typical halo-owl eye
Viral replication tubules	Yes	Yes
Endothelial cells	No	Yes
Inflammatory cells	No	Yes
Acute tubular injury	Rarely	Rarely
Interstitial inflammation	Focal to diffuse	Focal
Tubulitis	Mild to severe	Mild

Table 2.
Histologic features of CMV and polyoma BK viral lesions in transplanted kidney.

The challenging concepts of immune reconstitution injury and extensive inflammation in resolving BKN after reducing immunosuppression need further investigation [6].

3.6 Clinical presentation and management of BKN

3.6.1 Clinical presentation and prognosis

Various studies have indicated that different extents of BKN in the transplant may predict the clinical presentation and outcome of the disease [58, 60, 61].

In order to provide optimal diagnostic and prognostic information of BKN, the Banff working group on BKN proposed three clinically significant disease grades based on the severity of polyomavirus replication and the degree of interstitial fibrosis [47, 62, 63]. BK virus replication was defined as the histologic viral load, estimated by the % of virally infected epithelial cells detected by immunohistochemistry. It ranged from scattered SV-40-positive cells in BKN grade 1 to numerous in grades 2 and 3 (**Figures 12–14**). In addition to SV-40-positive cells, grade 3 is characterized by interstitial fibrosis, which is responsible for irreversible tissue injury leading to graft failure [5, 47, 62].

Disease grade may reflect the time of the diagnosis: BKN grade 1 was generally diagnosed in the first 5 months after transplantation, usually presenting with normal renal function and associated with a favorable outcome in 85–90% of cases. In contrast, grade 2 BKN was detected 6–12 months posttransplantation, characterized by elevated serum creatinine or acute graft injury leading to graft failure in 25% of cases. Finally, BKN grade 3 was usually detected more than 12 months after transplantation, also associated with worsening of kidney function and graft failure in 50% of cases (**Table 3**).

Since BKN has limited treatment options, the early detection of PVN has a major impact on the prognosis of the disease and therefore on allograft survival. Early diagnosis of PVN is difficult, because early BKN stage does not show any signs of systemic infection, proteinuria, or hematuria. Renal function may remain normal transiently, particularly when only the medulla is involved [5].

PVN disease grade	Viral load	Interstitial fibrosis	Renal function	Time of diagnosis after TX (months)	Favorable outcome (%)
Grade 1	Scattered SV-40-positive cells	No	Normal	4–5	85–90
Grade 2	Numerous	Less than 25%	Increased serum creatinine, renal failure	6–12	75
Grade 3	Numerous	More than 25%	Increased serum creatinine, acute renal failure	12	50

Table 3.
Characteristics of different BKN grades regarding viral load, chronic tissue injury-interstitial fibrosis, renal function, time of diagnosis after transplantation, and outcome.

3.6.2 Screening of PVN

To date, reduction of baseline immunosuppression remains the only potentially effective therapeutic strategy of BKN, but it is associated with an increased risk of rejection. It is considered that preemptive reduction of immunosuppression prior to the development of overt nephropathy might be beneficial [6, 51, 59]. Since unrecognized BKN diagnosed late after transplantation causes chronic tissue injury and graft failure, the goal of screening protocols and classification schemes of BKN is to characterize early disease grades that respond to therapeutic intervention and may heal without progressing to chronic graft injury.

The first step of viral reactivation shown in almost all patients is characterized by the detection of characteristic polyomavirus inclusion-bearing cells in the urine—decoy cells (**Figure 15**). Initial viruria may be followed by detection of BK virus in plasma and onset of BKN after a 6–12-week window in some patients but only in a minority (**Figure 16**) [51].

Current guidelines recommend a urinary cytology test in order to detect urinary decoy cells initially and then a plasma test by PCR if urinary decoy cells are consistently present [51]. While PVN is most commonly diagnosed in the first year after transplantation, urine screening at least every 3 months during the first 2 years and after antirejection treatment seems appropriate to cover the majority of PVN cases [51]. The cytology urine test is characterized by a high negative predictive value to rule out a diagnosis of BKN and reduce costs. In addition, a window between viral reactivation and BKN enables urine samples to be screened in time.

However, several studies have shown that only a variable number of patients with urinary shedding of virus progressed to BKN. Notably, BK viruria and even

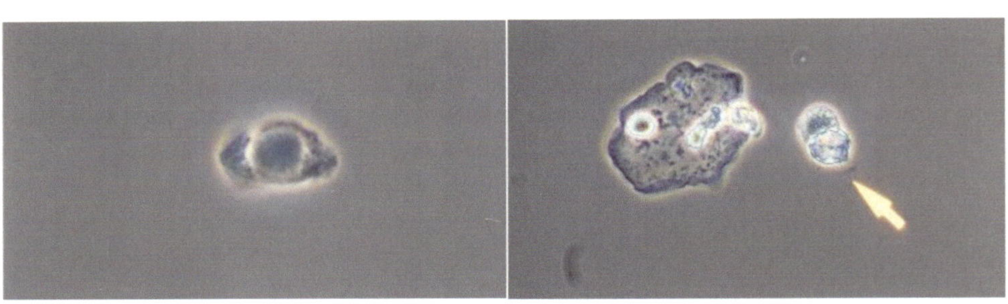

Figure 15.
Decoy cells in urine screening test.

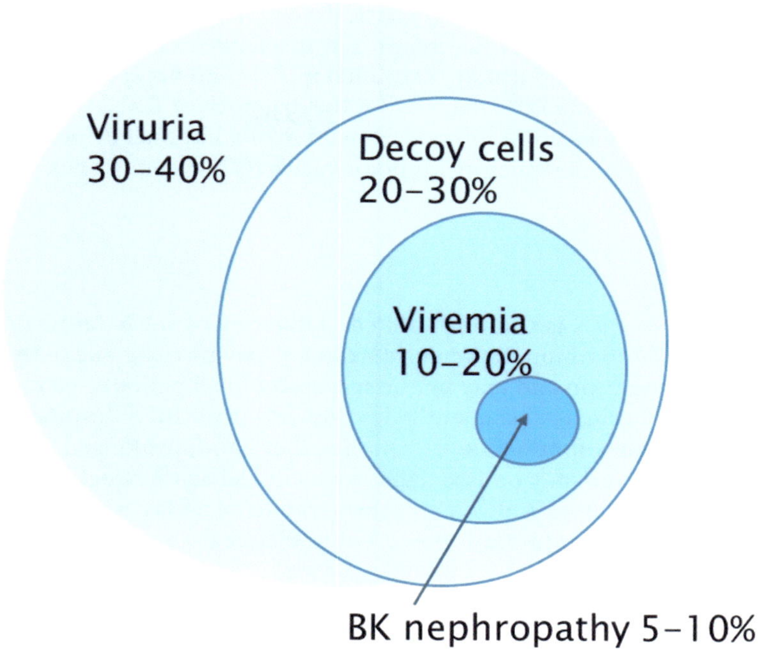

Figure 16.
Type and prevalence of BK virus (BKV) infections in kidney transplant recipients.

viremia may represent transient asymptomatic BK activation or may originate from extrarenal sites, usually along the lower urinary tract. In patients without biopsy-proven BKN, preemptive long-lasting reduction of immunosuppression could be potentially harmful due to increased risk of acute rejection [64].

3.6.3 Biomarkers of BKN

A plasma test by PCR detecting BK copies is currently the accepted biomarker for clinical application, although the exact range of viral load that would predict BKN cannot be defined. The majority of patients with more than 10,000 copies per ml DNA in 1 ml of plasma show BKN on renal biopsy, but some patients with hardly detectable BK virus copy numbers may have manifest BKN. Several studies have indicated that PCR-based BK viremia correlates only moderately well with the presence of BKN and severity of the intrarenal disease, ranging between 25 and 75% (**Figure 15**) [6, 57].

Several biomarkers had been proposed in order to enable noninvasive diagnosis of definitive BKN without the risk of renal biopsy; these include heat shock protein 90alfa, CXCL9, neutrophil gelatinase-associated lipocalin, urinary exosomal biomarkers, urinary VP1, and urinary Haufen [65–67].

Polyomavirus-Haufen are tight cast-like three-dimensional viral aggregates, detected by negative staining electron microscopy of a voided urine sample. Since polyomavirus-Haufen admixed with uromodulin is formed in the tubular lumens, they might specifically predict intrarenal disease, comparable to renal biopsy [68]. Recent studies have indicated that the titer of polyomavirus-Haufen tightly correlates with the degree of intrarenal polyomavirus replication, providing additional information on the severity of PVN [64]. The urinary polyomavirus-Haufen test may emerge as a sensitive and specific biomarker for intrarenal viral disease, with positive and negative predictive value higher than 90%. The limitations of this investigation include the relatively high cost, time-consuming procedure, and limited availability of electron microscopy in transplant centers.

BK virus VP1 mRNA and urinary exosomal miRNA biomarkers have been described as potential surrogate markers for the diagnosis of PVN, with high sensitivity and specificity for BKN [66, 67]. Detection of additional urine biomarkers not only offers additional strategies for noninvasive PVN diagnosis but might also predict graft outcome.

3.6.4 Treatment of BKN

Management of PVN is still very limited. Reduction of the baseline immunosuppression, as the common therapeutic strategy, may be risky due to the possibility of acute rejection and may not be successful in all patients. Namely, some patients with BK viremia subsequently develop definitive BKN despite preemptive reduction of immunosuppression [4]. On the other hand, prolonged reduction of immunosuppression may be associated with clinical acute rejection rates of 8–14% [5, 69]. Renal biopsy, although considered to be an invasive procedure, may provide additional information in order to diagnose concomitant vascular rejection.

Data concerning the frequency of concurrent PVN and rejection vary. Some authors consider inflammation to be part of immune reconstitution injury, with a very low risk of concomitant rejection, whereas others have diagnosed concurrent acute rejection in 10–15% of cases at the time of initial PVN diagnosis [6, 47, 63]. Additional corticosteroid treatment in patients with PVN and severe tubulointerstitial inflammation at the time of PVN diagnosis also remains controversial. Some authors believe that corticosteroid treatment interferes with efficient BK clearance from the graft although, on the other hand, it might decrease interstitial inflammation and subsequent interstitial fibrosis [59].

Biopsy-proven diagnosis of concurrent BKN and rejection reveals the therapeutic dilemma concerning treatment strategy. In some individual cases, concomitant biopsy-proven T-cell-mediated rejection and PVN on low immunosuppression have been efficiently treated with transient pulse immunosuppressive therapy [70]. On surveillance kidney biopsy, BK was cleared from the tissue, interstitial inflammation disappeared, and serum creatinine returned to the baseline level.

Many of the therapeutic agents, including leflunomide, quinolone, and cidofovir, have been involved in BKN treatment with undetermined antipolyomavirus effect. It was recently shown that intravenous immunoglobulins' (IV IGs) administration may be effective in the treatment of BK viremia and PVN in patients who have failed to respond to immunosuppression reduction and leflunomide therapy [71].

Successful resolution of BKN and BK clearance may be associated with the recipient's antiviral cell-mediated immune response. Recently, novel laboratory-based methods based on BK-directed cellular immunity and anti-BK T-cell phenotype have been introduced, such as ELISPOT assays, which might provide additional information in relation to the resolution of PVN [72–74].

4. Conclusions

KTRs receiving immunosuppressive regimes to prevent transplant rejection are at increased risk of opportunistic infections such as CMV and polyoma BK virus. In both viruses, reactivation of latent infection is the principal mechanism rather than de novo infection.

While reactivation of CMV infection is usually present with systemic infection, including fever, leukopenia, organ dysfunction, and viremia without invading renal graft, the most harmful presentation of BK infection reactivation includes BKN directly affecting the transplanted kidney.

Both CMV and BK infections commonly appear in the first year after transplantation, so screening protocols are very important in order to detect patients with increased risk of virus reactivation and early disease, and this should be started immediately after transplantation.

With systematically quantitative monitoring of CMV DNA in plasma, CMV viremia can be detected before the occurrence of symptomatic infection. Ganciclovir and valganciclovir are generally used to prevent or treat CMV.

For BKN screening, current guidelines recommend a urinary cytology test initially and then plasma DNA test by PCR if urinary decoy cells are consistently found.

The reduction of baseline immunosuppression is considered to be the common therapeutic strategy of BKN but is associated with increased risk of rejection. Since polyomavirus viruria and viremia can be observed without renal injury and BKN, a definite diagnosis of PVN must be confirmed by renal biopsy. In order to prevent BKN in viremic patients, preemptive reduction of immunosuppression prior to the development of overt nephropathy might be beneficial.

Careful detection and management of opportunistic infection enable better graft survival and quality of life in KTRs.

Acknowledgements

The authors would like to acknowledge Jerica Pleško, Karmen Wechtersbach, Živa Pipan Tkalec, Špela Borštnar, MD, and Matic Bošnjak, MD for their valuable help with providing figure material for this chapter. Professor Danica Galešić Ljubanović, MD PhD and Petar Šenjug, MD provided figures of CMV nephritis.

Conflict of interest

Authors declare no conflict of interest.

Author details

Večerić-Haler Željka* and Kojc Nika
Department of Nephrology, University Medical Centre Ljubljana, Ljubljana, Slovenia

*Address all correspondence to: zeljka.vecerichaler@kclj.si

References

[1] Fishman JA. Infection in solid-organ transplant recipients. The New England Journal of Medicine. 2007;**357**(25):2601-2614

[2] Kaminski H, Fishman JA. The cell biology of cytomegalovirus: Implications for transplantation. American Journal of Transplantation. 2016;**16**(8):2254-2269

[3] Ramanan P, Razonable RR. Cytomegalovirus infections in solid organ transplantation: A review. Infection & Chemotherapy. 2013;**45**(3):260-271

[4] Schaub S, Hirsch HH, Dickenmann M, Steiger J, Mihatsch MJ, Hopfer H, et al. Reducing immunosuppression preserves allograft function in presumptive and definitive polyomavirus-associated nephropathy. American Journal of Transplantation. 2010;**10**(12):2615-2623

[5] Nickeleit V, Nickeleit V, Singh HK, Randhawa P. The banff working group classification of definitive polyomavirus nephropathy: Morphologic definitions and clinical correlations. Journal of the American Society of Nephrology. 2018;**29**(2):680-693

[6] Menter T, Mayr M, Schaub S, Mihatsch MJ, Hirsch HH, Hopfer H. Pathology of resolving polyomavirus-associated nephropathy. American Journal of Transplantation. 2013;**13**(6):1474-1483

[7] Griffiths P, Baraniak I, Reeves M. The pathogenesis of human cytomegalovirus. The Journal of Pathology. 2015;**235**(2):288-297

[8] Giakoustidis D, Antoniadis A, Fouzas I, Sklavos A, Giakoustidis A, Ouzounidis N, et al. Prevalence and clinical impact of cytomegalovirus infection and disease in renal transplantation: Ten years of experience in a single center. Transplantation Proceedings. 2012;**44**(9):2715-2717

[9] Crough T, Khanna R. Immunobiology of human cytomegalovirus: From bench to bedside. Clinical Microbiology Reviews. 2009;**22**(1):76-98, Table of Contents

[10] Dupont L, Reeves MB. Cytomegalovirus latency and reactivation: Recent insights into an age old problem. Reviews in Medical Virology. 2016;**26**(2):75-89

[11] Han SH. Immunological prediction of cytomegalovirus (CMV) replication risk in solid organ transplantation recipients: Approaches for regulating the targeted anti-CMV prevention strategies. Infection & Chemotherapy. 2017;**49**(3):161-175

[12] Martin-Gandul C, Mueller NJ, Pascual M, Manuel O. The impact of infection on chronic allograft dysfunction and allograft survival after solid organ transplantation. American Journal of Transplantation. 2015;**15**(12):3024-3040

[13] Ljungman P, Griffiths P, Paya C. Definitions of cytomegalovirus infection and disease in transplant recipients. Clinical Infectious Diseases. 2002;**34**(8):1094-1097

[14] Lumbreras C, Manuel O, Len O, ten Berge IJ, Sgarabotto D, Hirsch HH. Cytomegalovirus infection in solid organ transplant recipients. Clinical Microbiology and Infection. 2014;**20**(Suppl 7):19-26

[15] Ross SA, Novak Z, Pati S, Boppana SB. Overview of the diagnosis of cytomegalovirus infection. Infectious Disorders Drug Targets. 2011;**11**(5):466-474

[16] Naumnik B, Małyszko J, Chyczewski L, Kovalchuk O, Myśliwiec M.

Comparison of serology assays and polymerase chain reaction for the monitoring of active cytomegalovirus infection in renal transplant recipients. Transplantation Proceedings. 2007;**39**(9):2748-2750

[17] Wong NA. Gastrointestinal pathology in transplant patients. Histopathology. 2015;**66**(4):467-479

[18] Vichot AA, Formica RN, Moeckel GW. Cytomegalovirus glomerulopathy and cytomegalovirus interstitial nephritis on sequential transplant kidney biopsies. American Journal of Kidney Diseases. 2014;**63**(3):536-539

[19] Agrawal V, Gupta RK, Jain M, Prasad N, Sharma RK. Polyomavirus nephropathy and cytomegalovirus nephritis in renal allograft recipients. Indian Journal of Pathology & Microbiology. 2010;**53**(4):672-675

[20] Joshi K, Nada R, Radotra BD, Jha V, Sakhuja V. Pathological spectrum of cytomegalovirus infection of renal allograft recipients—An autopsy study from North India. Indian Journal of Pathology & Microbiology. 2004;**47**(3):327-332

[21] Battegay EJ, Mihatsch MJ, Mazzucchelli L, Zollinger HU, Gudat F, Thiel G, et al. Cytomegalovirus and kidney. Clinical Nephrology. 1988;**30**(5):239-247

[22] Rane S, Nada R, Minz M, Sakhuja V, Joshi K. Spectrum of cytomegalovirus-induced renal pathology in renal allograft recipients. Transplantation Proceedings. 2012;**44**(3):713-716

[23] Reinke P, Fietze E, Ode-Hakim S, Prösch S, Lippert J, Ewert R, et al. Late-acute renal allograft rejection and symptomless cytomegalovirus infection. Lancet. 1994;**344**(8939-8940):1737-1738

[24] El-Zimaity H, Choi WT, Lauwers GY, Riddell R. The differential diagnosis of *Helicobacter pylori* negative gastritis. Virchows Archiv. 2018;**473**(5):533-550

[25] You DM, Johnson MD. Cytomegalovirus infection and the gastrointestinal tract. Current Gastroenterology Reports. 2012;**14**(4):334-342

[26] Agaimy A, Mudter J, Märkl B, Chetty R. Cytomegalovirus infection presenting as isolated inflammatory polyps of the gastrointestinal tract. Pathology. 2011;**43**(5):440-446

[27] Kambham N, Vij R, Cartwright CA, Longacre T. Cytomegalovirus infection in steroid-refractory ulcerative colitis: A case-control study. The American Journal of Surgical Pathology. 2004;**28**(3):365-373

[28] Ljungman P. CMV infections after hematopoietic stem cell transplantation. Bone Marrow Transplantation. 2008;**42**(Suppl 1):S70-S72

[29] Lemonovich TL, Watkins RR. Update on cytomegalovirus infections of the gastrointestinal system in solid organ transplant recipients. Current Infectious Disease Reports. 2012;**14**(1):33-40

[30] Lawlor G, Moss AC. Cytomegalovirus in inflammatory bowel disease: Pathogen or innocent bystander? Inflammatory Bowel Diseases. 2010;**16**(9):1620-1627

[31] Zidar N, Ferkolj I, Tepeš K, Štabuc B, Kojc N, Uršič T, et al. Diagnosing cytomegalovirus in patients with inflammatory bowel disease—By immunohistochemistry or polymerase chain reaction? Virchows Archiv. 2015;**466**(5):533-539

[32] Fehr T, Cippà PE, Mueller NJ. Cytomegalovirus post kidney transplantation: Prophylaxis versus pre-emptive therapy? Transplant International. 2015;**28**(12):1351-1356

[33] Tomažič J. Preprečevanje in zdravljenje okužb, povzročenih z virusom citomegalije, pri presaditvah čvrstih organov. Zdravstveni Vestnik. 2011;**80**:285-292

[34] Kır O, Zeytinoğlu A, Arda B, Yılmaz M, Aşçı G, Töz H. Impact of prophylaxis vs pre-emptive approach for cytomegalovirus infection in kidney transplant recipients. Transplantation Proceedings. 2017;**49**(3):537-540

[35] Kotton CN, Kumar D, Caliendo AM, Asberg A, Chou S, Danziger-Isakov L, et al. Updated international consensus guidelines on the management of cytomegalovirus in solid-organ transplantation. Transplantation. 2013;**96**(4):333-360

[36] Večerić-Haler Ž, Bizjak B, Romozi K, Arnol M. Expanded valganciclovir prophylaxis in kidney transplant recipients is associated with lower incidence of cytomegalovirus infection. Clinical Nephrology. 2017;**88**(13):126-130

[37] Xin W, Hui Y, Xiaodong Z, Xiangli C, hihui W, Lihong L. Effectiveness of valganciclovir 900mg versus 450mg for cytomegalovirus prophylaxis in renal transplantation: A systematic review and meta-analysis. Journal of Pharmacy & Pharmaceutical Sciences. 2017;**20**(0):168-183

[38] Biron KK. Antiviral drugs for cytomegalovirus diseases. Antiviral Research. 2006;**71**(2-3):154-163

[39] Davis CL. The prevention of cytomegalovirus disease in renal transplantation. American Journal of Kidney Diseases. 1990;**16**(3):175-188

[40] Singh N. Preemptive therapy versus universal prophylaxis with ganciclovir for cytomegalovirus in solid organ transplant recipients. Clinical Infectious Diseases. 2001;**32**(5):742-751

[41] Lee H, Park KH, Ryu JH, Choi AR, Yu JH, Lim J, et al. Cytomegalovirus (CMV) immune monitoring with ELISPOT and QuantiFERON-CMV assay in seropositive kidney transplant recipients. PLoS One. 2017;**12**(12):e0189488

[42] Tan BH. Cytomegalovirus treatment. Current Treatment Options in Infectious Diseases. 2014;**6**(3):256-270

[43] Aslani HR, Ziaie S, Salamzadeh J, Zaheri S, Samadian F, Mastoor-Tehrani S. Incidence of ganciclovir resistance in CMV-positive renal transplant recipients and its association with UL97 gene mutations. Iranian Journal of Pharmaceutical Research. 2017;**16**(2):805-810

[44] Cintra-Cabrera M, Suárez-Benjumea A, Bernal-Blanco G, González-Roncero FM, Toapanta-Gaibor NG, Súñer-Poblet M, et al. Resistant cytomegalovirus infection after renal transplantation: Literature review. Transplantation Proceedings. 2018;**50**(2):575-577

[45] Gardiner BJ, Chow JK, Price LL, Nierenberg NE, Kent DM, Snydman DR. Role of secondary prophylaxis with valganciclovir in the prevention of recurrent cytomegalovirus disease in solid organ transplant recipients. Clinical Infectious Diseases. 2017;**65**(12):2000-2007

[46] Dalianis T, Hirsch HH. Human polyomaviruses in disease and cancer. Virology. 2013;**437**(2):63-72

[47] Nickeleit V, Singh HK. Polyomaviruses and disease: Is there more to know than viremia and viruria? Current Opinion in Organ Transplantation. 2015;**20**(3):348-358

[48] Kenan DJ, Mieczkowski PA, Burger-Calderon R, Singh HK, Nickeleit V. The oncogenic potential of BK-polyomavirus

is linked to viral integration into the human genome. The Journal of Pathology. 2015;**237**(3):379-389

[49] Burger-Calderon R, Madden V, Hallett RA, Gingerich AD, Nickeleit V, Webster-Cyriaque J. Replication of oral BK virus in human salivary gland cells. Journal of Virology. 2014;**88**(1):559-573

[50] Coursaget P, Samimi M, Nicol JT, Gardair C, Touzé A. Human Merkel cell polyomavirus: Virological background and clinical implications. APMIS. 2013;**121**(8):755-769

[51] Masutani K. Current problems in screening, diagnosis and treatment of polyomavirus BK nephropathy. Nephrology (Carlton, Vic.). 2014;**19**(Suppl 3):11-16

[52] Sharma SG, Nickeleit V, Herlitz LC, de Gonzalez AK, Stokes MB, Singh HK, et al. BK polyoma virus nephropathy in the native kidney. Nephrology, Dialysis, Transplantation. 2013;**28**(3):620-631

[53] van der Bij A, Betjes M, Weening J, Cornelissen J, Mes T, Osterhaus A, et al. BK virus nephropathy in an immunodeficient patient with chronic lymphocytic leukemia. Journal of Clinical Virology. 2009;**45**(4):341-344

[54] Hashim F, Rehman S, Gregg JA, Dharnidharka VR. Ureteral stent placement increases the risk for developing BK viremia after kidney transplantation. Journal of Transplantation. 2014;**2014**:459747

[55] Hirsch HH, Brennan DC, Drachenberg CB, Ginevri F, Gordon J, Limaye AP, et al. Polyomavirus-associated nephropathy in renal transplantation: Interdisciplinary analyses and recommendations. Transplantation. 2005;**79**(10):1277-1286

[56] Hirsch HH, Babel N, Comoli P, Friman V, Ginevri F, Jardine A, et al. European perspective on human polyomavirus infection, replication and disease in solid organ transplantation. Clinical Microbiology and Infection. 2014;**20**(Suppl 7):74-88

[57] Hirsch HH, Randhawa P, AIDCo P. BK polyomavirus in solid organ transplantation. American Journal of Transplantation. 2013;**13**Suppl 4:179-188

[58] Sis B, Mengel M, Haas M, Colvin RB, Halloran PF, Racusen LC, et al. Banff '09 meeting report: Antibody mediated graft deterioration and implementation of banff working groups. American Journal of Transplantation. 2010;**10**(3):464-471

[59] Schaub S, Mayr M, Egli A, Binggeli S, Descoeudres B, Steiger J, et al. Transient allograft dysfunction from immune reconstitution in a patient with polyoma BK-virus-associated nephropathy. Nephrology, Dialysis, Transplantation. 2007;**22**(8):2386-2390

[60] Drachenberg RC, Drachenberg CB, Papadimitriou JC, Ramos E, Fink JC, Wali R, et al. Morphological spectrum of polyoma virus disease in renal allografts: Diagnostic accuracy of urine cytology. American Journal of Transplantation. 2001;**1**(4):373-381

[61] Nishi S. Polyomavirus nephropathy—Recent pathological diagnostic problems and the report from the 2011 Banff meeting. Clinical Transplantation. 2012;**26**(Suppl 24):9-12

[62] Haas M, Sis B, Racusen LC, Solez K, Glotz D, Colvin RB, et al. Banff 2013 meeting report: Inclusion of c4d-negative antibody-mediated rejection and antibody-associated arterial lesions. American Journal of Transplantation. 2014;**14**(2):272-283

[63] Nickeleit V, Mihatsch MJ. Polyomavirus allograft nephropathy and concurrent acute rejection: A diagnostic and therapeutic challenge.

American Journal of Transplantation. 2004;**4**(5):838-839

[64] Singh HK, Reisner H, Derebail VK, Kozlowski T, Nickeleit V. Polyomavirus nephropathy: Quantitative urinary polyomavirus-Haufen testing accurately predicts the degree of intrarenal viral disease. Transplantation. 2015;**99**(3):609-615

[65] Singh HK, Andreoni KA, Madden V, True K, Detwiler R, Weck K, et al. Presence of urinary Haufen accurately predicts polyomavirus nephropathy. Journal of the American Society of Nephrology. 2009;**20**(2):416-427

[66] Dadhania D, Snopkowski C, Muthukumar T, Lee J, Ding R, Sharma VK, et al. Noninvasive prognostication of polyomavirus BK virus-associated nephropathy. Transplantation. 2013;**96**(2):131-138

[67] Kim MH, Lee YH, Seo JW, Moon H, Kim JS, Kim YG, et al. Urinary exosomal viral microRNA as a marker of BK virus nephropathy in kidney transplant recipients. PLoS One. 2017;**12**(12):e0190068

[68] Singh HK, Donna Thompson B, Nickeleit V. Viral Haufen are urinary biomarkers of polyomavirus nephropathy: New diagnostic strategies utilizing negative staining electron microscopy. Ultrastructural Pathology. 2009;**33**(5):222-235

[69] Sood P, Senanayake S, Sujeet K, Medipalli R, Zhu YR, Johnson CP, et al. Management and outcome of BK viremia in renal transplant recipients: A prospective single-center study. Transplantation. 2012;**94**(8):814-821

[70] Kojc N, Aleš Rigler A, Mlinšek G, Kovač D, Ferluga D, Arnol M. Outcome of polyomavirus nephropathy in renal transplant patients: A single-center experience. Clinical Nephrology. 2017;**88**(13):109-114

[71] Vu D, Shah T, Ansari J, Naraghi R, Min D. Efficacy of intravenous immunoglobulin in the treatment of persistent BK viremia and BK virus nephropathy in renal transplant recipients. Transplantation Proceedings. 2015;**47**(2):394-398

[72] Prosser SE, Orentas RJ, Jurgens L, Cohen EP, Hariharan S. Recovery of BK virus large T-antigen-specific cellular immune response correlates with resolution of bk virus nephritis. Transplantation. 2008;**85**(2):185-192

[73] Mueller K, Schachtner T, Sattler A, Meier S, Friedrich P, Trydzenskaya H, et al. BK-VP3 as a new target of cellular immunity in BK virus infection. Transplantation. 2011;**91**(1):100-107

[74] Schachtner T, Müller K, Stein M, Diezemann C, Sefrin A, Babel N, et al. BK virus-specific immunity kinetics: A predictor of recovery from polyomavirus BK-associated nephropathy. American Journal of Transplantation. 2011;**11**(11):2443-2452

Chapter 4

Antibody Mediated Rejection in Kidney Transplant Recipients

Nika Kojc and Željka Večerić Haler

Abstract

Antibody mediated rejection (ABMR) presents a significant challenge for long term graft survival in kidney transplantation. New technologies, including genomic studies and assays to detect and define donor-specific antibodies, have provided important insights into the pathophysiology and diagnosis of ABMR. Unfortunately, this progress has not yet translated into better outcomes for patients, as in the absence of a drug able to suppress antibody generation by plasma cells, available therapies can only slow down graft destruction. This chapter reviews the current understanding of ABMR, and details its diagnosis, and treatments, both those established in current routine clinical practice and those on the horizon.

Keywords: antibody mediated rejection, humoral rejection, kidney rejection, kidney transplantation, kidney transplant rejection, donor specific antibodies

1. Introduction

Antibody-mediated rejection (ABMR), also termed humoral rejection, is one of the most important causes of allograft dysfunction and loss accounting for up to 76% of death-censored graft failures beyond the first year of transplantation [1, 2]. According to current evidence, B cell and plasma cell activation results in the generation of donor-specific antibodies (DSAs), which bind to human leukocyte antigen (HLA) or non-HLA molecules expressed on endothelial cells within the renal allograft [3].

ABMR often represents a pathological spectrum that co-exists with T-cell-mediated rejection [3]. Active (acute) ABMR is characterized by serological evidence of DSA, peritubular capillaritis, glomerulitis, cellular necrosis, thrombotic microangiopathy, and a relatively rapid decline in allograft function. The response to currently available therapies is often favorable. Chronic ABMR, on the other hand, is characterized by transplant glomerulopathy, a distinct pathophysiological process resulting from a repetitive pattern of thrombotic events and inflammatory changes that lead to endothelial cell injury and allograft matrix remodeling. It usually results in a slow and progressive decline in renal function, unlikely to be reversed by current therapeutic strategies [3, 4].

2. Pathogenesis

In the 1960 Kissmeyer et al. [5] were the first to observe the deleterious impact of allo-antibodies in kidney grafts. Since then great advances have

IntechOpen

occurred in solid organ transplantation. Nowadays, it is believed that immunologic reactions associated with ABMR can be triggered by circulating antibodies against donor HLA, non-HLA or ABO antigens, i.e. donor specific antibodies (DSAs) [6].

DSAs are most commonly directed against human leukocyte antigen (HLA)/ major-histocompatibility-complex (MHC) class I and II antigens [7]. HLA class I antigens are expressed on all nucleated cells, whereas HLA class II antigens are restricted to antigen-presenting cells (B lymphocytes, dendritic cells) and endothelial cells [8]. In addition to DSAs existing prior to transplant due to recipient sensitization (pregnancy, blood transfusions, and previous transplantation), it has been realized that they can emerge at any time after transplant, thus mediating allograft injury [9, 10]. These *de novo* DSAs are different in their pathogenicity. Those directed against class II HLA are associated with a worse prognosis than DSAs against class I HLA [10].

However, the antibodies can also be directed against other donor specific antigens such as MHC-class I-related chain A (MICA) antigens, MHC-class I-related chain B (MICB) antigens, platelet-specific antigens, molecules of the renin-angiotensin pathway, and polymorphisms involving chemokines and their receptors [11–13]. MICA antigens are expressed on endothelial cells, dendritic cells, fibroblasts, epithelial cells, and many tumors, but not on peripheral-blood lymphocytes [12].

The major mechanism involved in antibody-mediated kidney injury is activation of the classical complement pathway by the binding of DSA to HLA and subsequent binding of the C1 complex, which ultimately leads to formation of the membrane attack complex (C5b-C9) (**Figure 1**) [14, 15].

This leads to activation of polymorphonuclear inflammatory cells, NK cell and monocyte recruitment and inflammation, as well as activation of the coagulation cascade, which in turn leads to widespread microvascular injury evident as peritubular capillaritis, glomerulitis and microvascular thrombosis. B-cell responses against MHC antigens are T-cell dependent and require the involvement of antigen-presenting cells and costimulatory molecules such as CD40 ligand or soluble interleukins. These responses take 2–3 weeks to develop and lead to immunologic memory, allowing a more efficient antibody response upon repeat stimulation. Eventually transplant glomerulopathy develops (chronic phase) due to recurrent injury and repair with glomerular basement

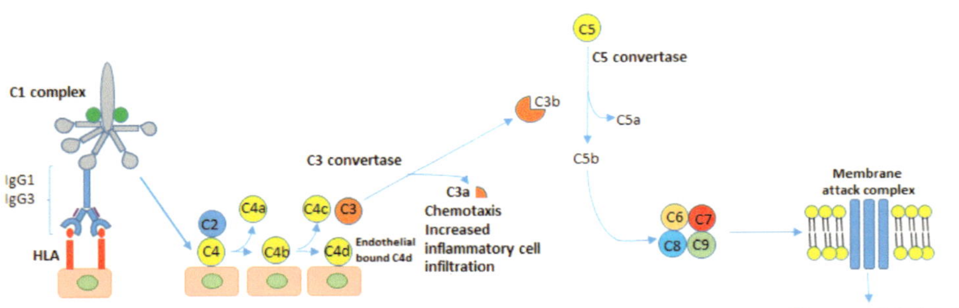

Figure 1.
Activation of classical complement pathway in ABMR in renal transplant recipients. Following binding of DSA to the vascular endothelium of kidney allograft, the C1 complex activates the serine esterases C1s and C1r, resulting in the cleavage of C4, deposition of C4d, and the assembly of the classical pathway C3 convertase. C3 convertase cleaves C3 into C3a, a potent pro-inflammatory mediator, and C3b, which propagates the complement cascade and leads to the formation of the pro-inflammatory mediator C5a and the membrane attack complex (C5b-C9). For more details, see Stegall et al. [15] ABMR-antibody-mediated rejection; DSA-donor-specific antibody; HLA-human leukocyte antigen.

membrane remodeling, mesangial matrix expansion, capillary obliteration, foot process effacement [15]. Microcirculation remodeling at the level of peritubular capillaries progresses to interstitial fibrosis and tubular atrophy causing allograft failure.

3. Diagnostic criteria for antibody mediated rejection

3.1 Histopathological features

By light microscopy, active antibody mediated rejection is characterized by 3 types of tissue injury: acute tubular injury, microcirculation inflammation with neutrophils and mononuclear cells in glomeruli and peritubular capillaries, and fibrinoid necrosis of arteries (**Figure 2**) [14].

Acute tubular injury includes loss of brush borders, thinning of tubular epithelial cells cytoplasm, shedding of tubular epithelium, and focal loss of nuclei (**Figure 3**). Focal necrosis of tubules can be found in minority of cases. In addition to oedema without significant interstitial infiltrate, proximal tubules express HLA-DR (**Figure 4**). Microcirculation inflammation with neutrophils and mononuclear cells in glomeruli and peritubular capillaries appears as glomerulitis and peritubular capillaritis. Glomerular capillaries are dilated and filled with swollen endothelial cells and inflammatory cells (**Figure 5**). In severe cases, glomerular capillary thrombosis can be detected (**Figure 6**). In glomerular injury due to ABMR usually predominates macrophages which express CD68 and neutrophils.

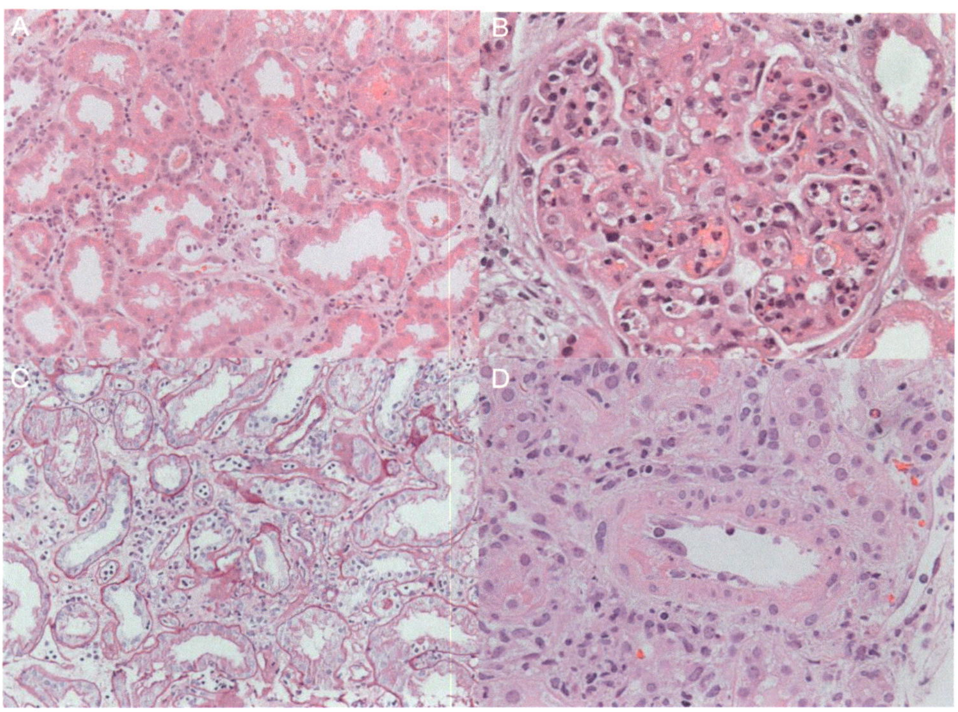

Figure 2.
Features of active antibody mediated rejection: Acute tubular injury [(A) hematoxylin-eosin stain (HE), 200×], microcirculation inflammation with neutrophils and mononuclear cells in glomeruli-glomerulitis [(B) HE, 400×] and peritubular capillaries-peritubular capillaritis [(C) HE, 200×], and fibrinoid necrosis of artery [(D) HE, 200×].

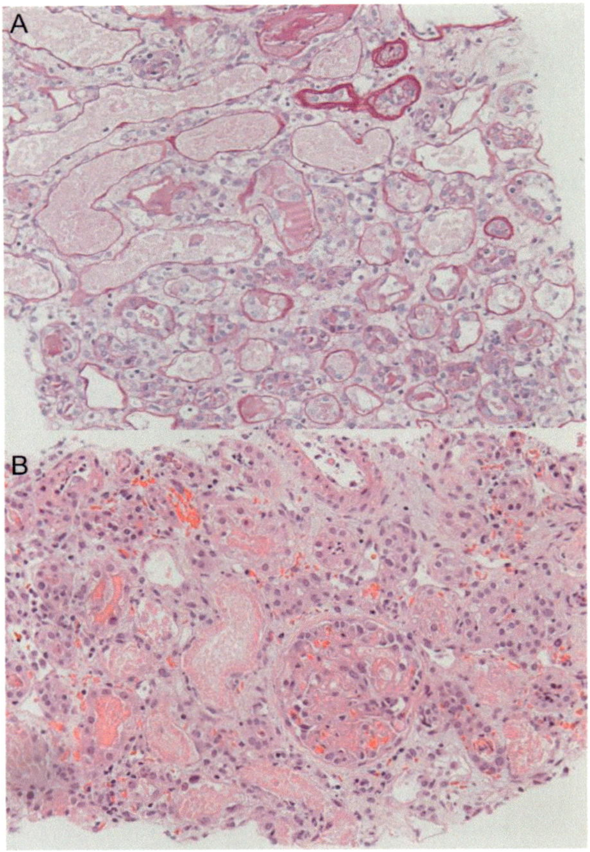

Figure 3.
Acute tubular injury/necrosis accompanied by interstitial edema in active antibody mediated rejection [(A) periodic-acid Schiff (PAS), 100×]. Acute tubular injury/necrosis and glomerular capillary necrosis [(B) HE, 100×].

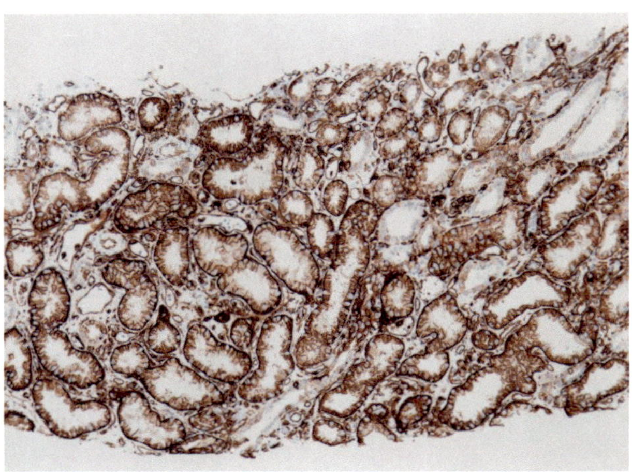

Figure 4.
Diffuse HLA-DR positivity in proximal tubules in active antibody mediated rejection (immunohistochemistry, HLA-DR, 100×).

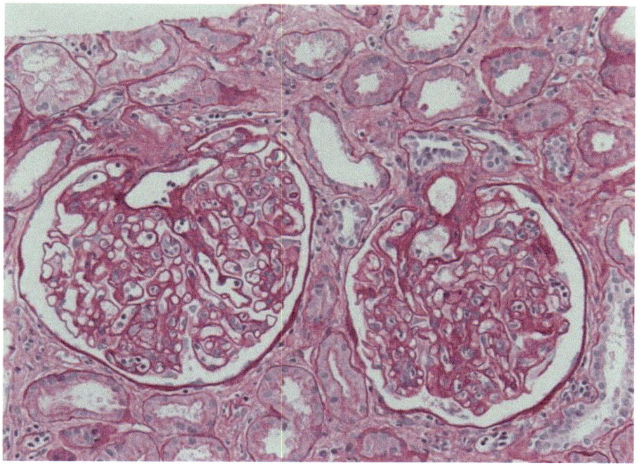

Figure 5.
Focal glomerulitis in active antibody mediated rejection-Banff score g3. Dilated glomerular capillaries are filled with swollen endothelial cells and inflammatory cells (PAS, 200×).

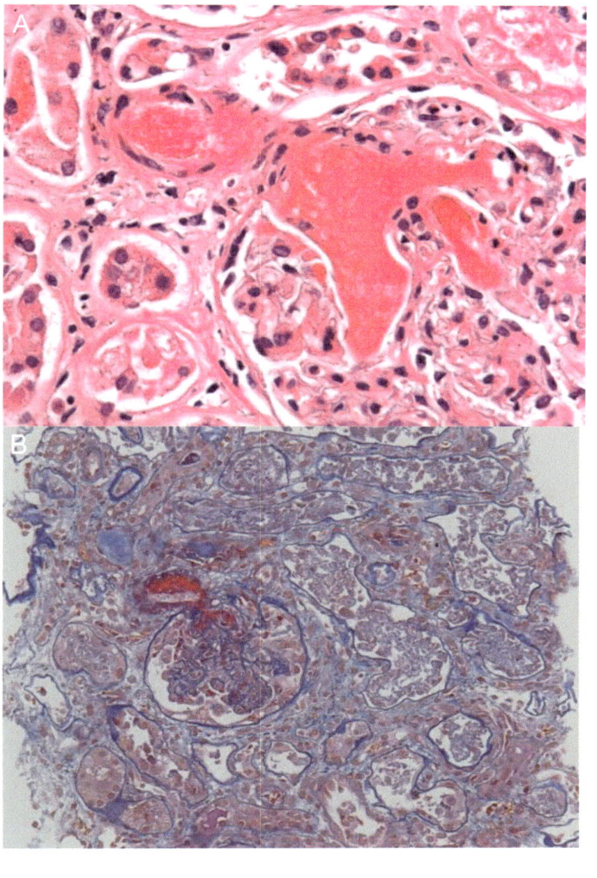

Figure 6.
Glomerular capillary thrombosis [(A) HE, 400×)] and fibrinoid necrosis of hilar arteriole [(B) trichrome stain, 200×)] in severe active antibody mediated rejection.

Cortical peritubular capillaries are dilated and filled with numerous inflammatory cells and sometimes focal interstitial hemorrhages are found (**Figure** 7). Presence of neutrophils in dilated peritubular capillaries may be associated with class I DSA and hyperacute rejection. Immunohistochemistry and immunofluorescence revealed diffuse linear positivity of C4d along peritubular capillaries in the

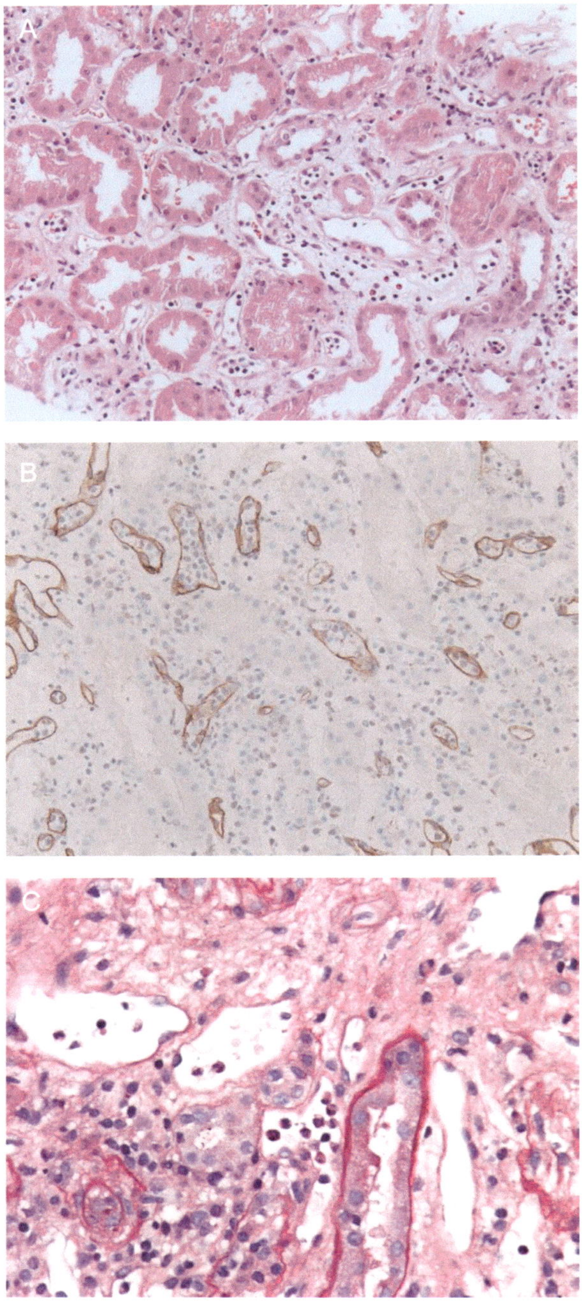

Figure 7.
Diffuse peritubular capillaritis in active antibody mediated rejection-Banff score ptc3 [(A and B) HE and immunohistochemistry, C4d, 200×)]. Neutrophils in peritubular capillaries in severe active antibody mediated rejection [(C) HE, 400×].

cortex and medulla (**Figure 8**). Dilated vascular spaces in the area between cortex and medulla should not be assessed as peritubular capillaritis, since those vascular spaces represent increased turnover between cortex and medulla not related to

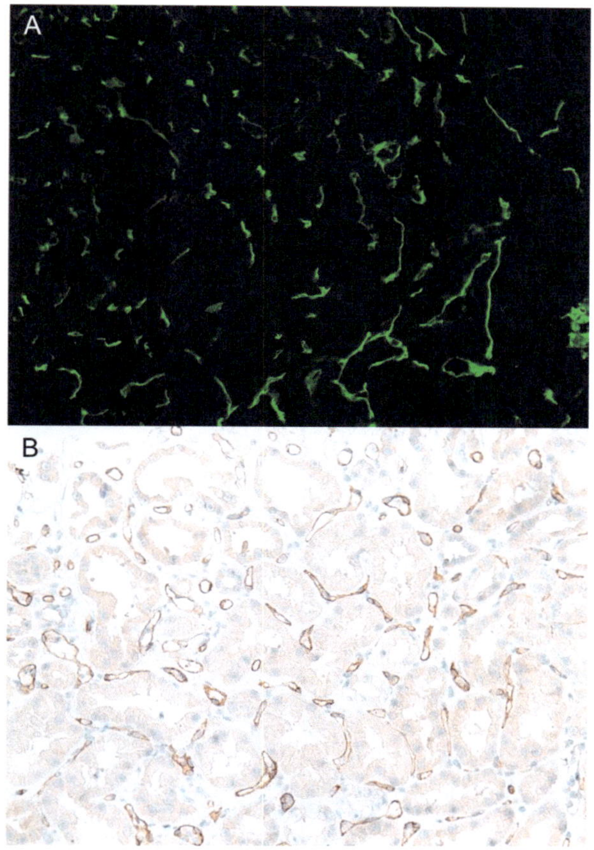

Figure 8.
Diffuse C4d positivity in active antibody mediated rejection (Banff score C4d 3) by immunofluorescence [(A) 200×] and immunohistochemistry [(B) 200×].

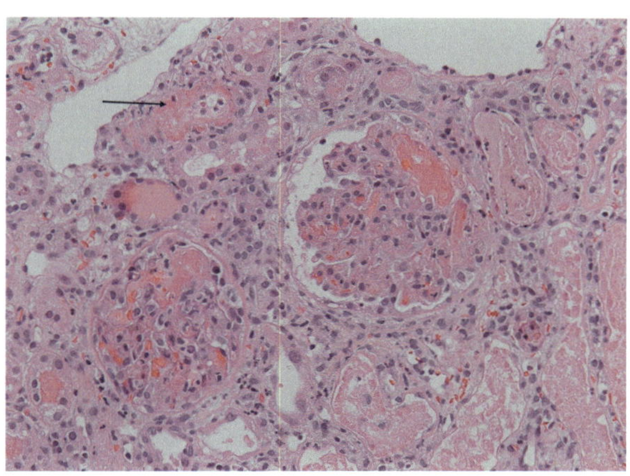

Figure 9.
Fibrinoid necrosis in small interlobular artery-Banff score v3 in severe active antibody mediated rejection (arrow). Glomerular capillary thrombosis and acute tubular necrosis are also seen (HE, 200×).

rejection. Interstitial oedema and hemorrhage may be prominent. B cells can be found in aggregates, and plasma cells can be detected, but interstitial infiltrate does not fulfill criteria for T-cell mediated rejection.

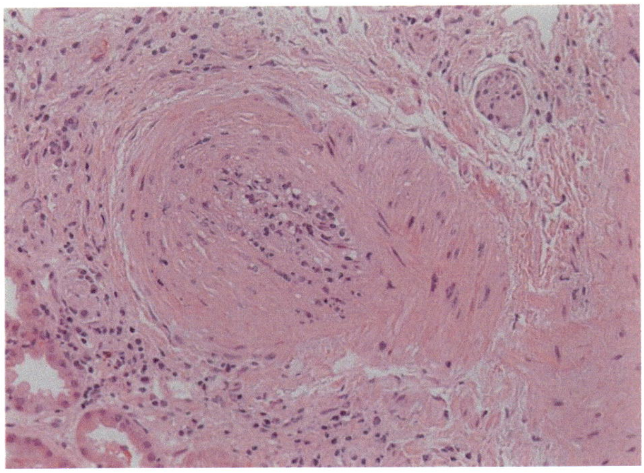

Figure 10.
Chronic active vascular rejection with intimal endarteritis and intimal fibrosis. HE, 200×.

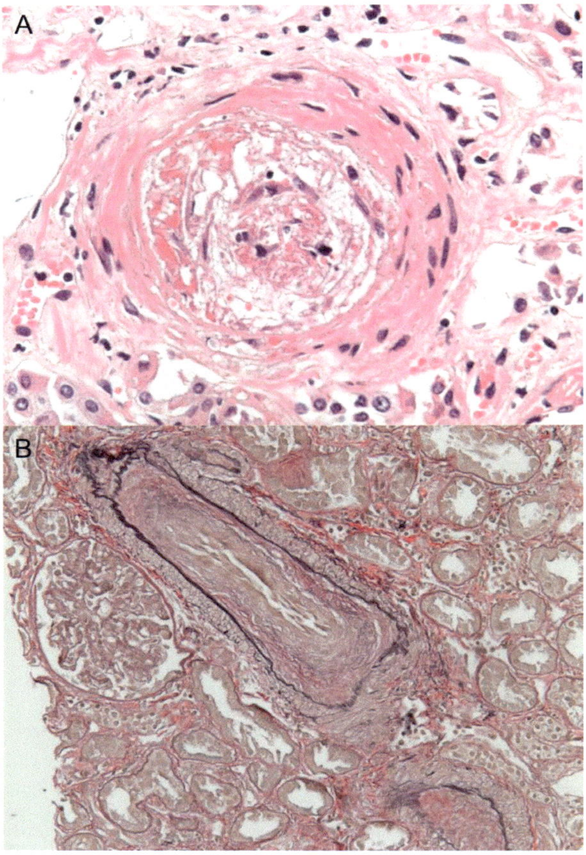

Figure 11.
Acute vascular thrombotic microangiopathy in active antibody mediated rejection [(A) HE, 200×]. Chronic glomerular and vascular thrombotic microangiopathy in chronic active antibody mediated rejection [(B) Weigert stain (W), 100×].

In about 25% of cases with ABMR, small interlobular arteries show myocyte necrosis, fragmentation of elastica, and accumulation of eosinophilic material termed fibrinoid necrosis (**Figure 9**). There is usually only scant mononuclear infiltrate in the intima and adventitia. Some arteries may show transmural arterial inflammation without fibrinoid necrosis reminiscent of T-cell mediated vascular rejection (**Figure 10**). Whether the cellular component of

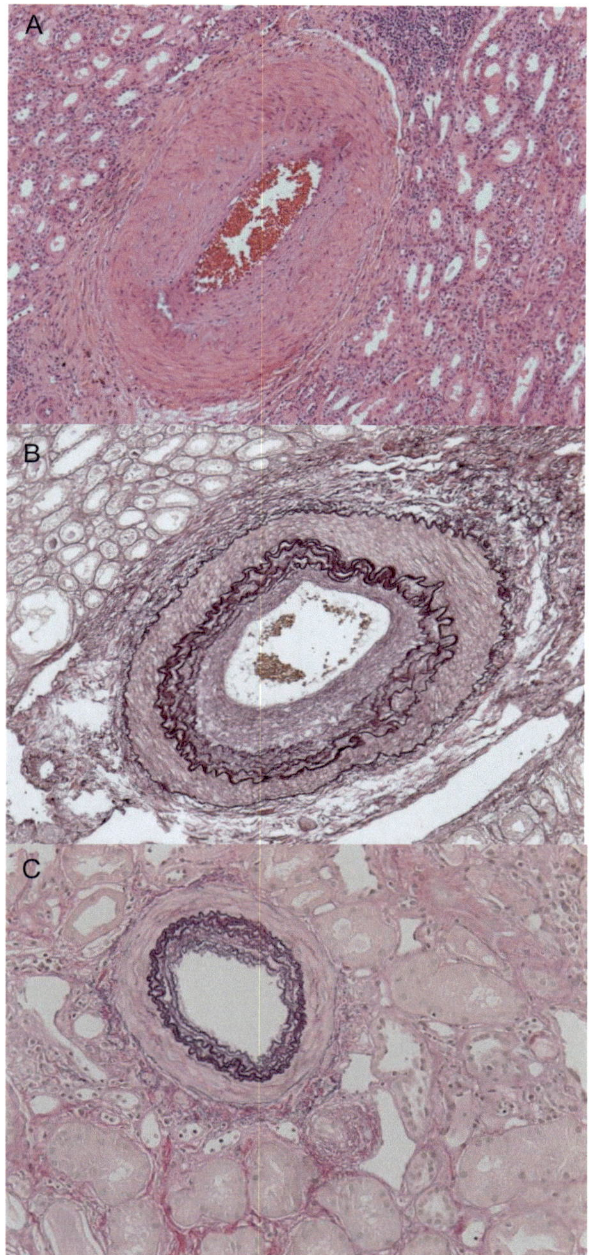

Figure 12.
Chronic burn out vascular rejection without intimal infiltrate in arcuate artery-Banff score cv3 [(A) HE, 100×]. Intimal fibrosis due to chronic rejection is superimposed on fibroelastic lamelation associated with arterial hypertension [(B) W, 100×]. Artery with elastic duplication due to arterial hypertension without rejection [(C) W, 100×].

transplant endarteritis in ABMR is different from that due to T-cell mediated rejection is not apparent. Arterial thrombosis is uncommon. However, acute ABMR may also manifest as TMA affecting glomerular and vascular endothelium (**Figure 11**). TMA is characterized by bloodless glomeruli with swollen endothelium and mucoid intimal thickening and trapped red cells in the vessel walls.

Over time, active ABMR usually transform to chronic ABMR with different levels of activity. Arterial lesions progress to intimal fibrosis with neomedia formation and progressive narrowing of vascular lumen (**Figure 12**) leading to chronic transplant changes—widespread interstitial fibrosis and tubular atrophy. In addition, chronic microvasculature changes appeared, including glomerular and peritubular capillaries. At the beginning, chronic glomerular lesions are visible only by EM as neolamina in glomerular capillary loops (**Figure 13**), which may progress to double contour formation and mesangial interposition seen by light microscopy (**Figure 14**). Peritubular capillaries electron micrograph revealed basement membrane multilamelation consistent with chronic ABMR (**Figure 15**) [14].

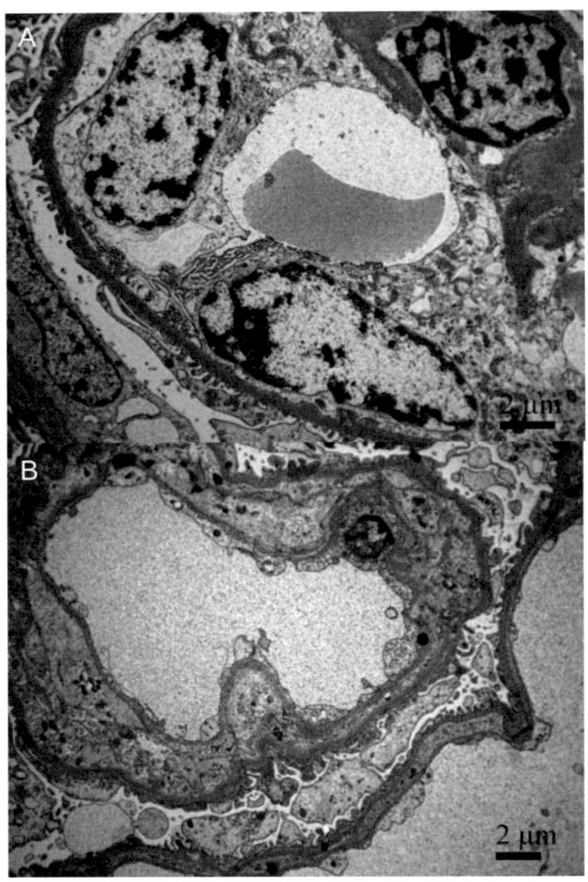

Figure 13.
Swollen endothelial cells in early glomerular thrombotic microangiopathy due to severe active antibody mediated rejection. Glomerular basement membrane appears normal (A). Subendothelial widening with oedema and neolamina formation in early chronic active antibody mediated rejection seen only by electron microscopy-Banff score cg1a [(B), all electron micrographs].

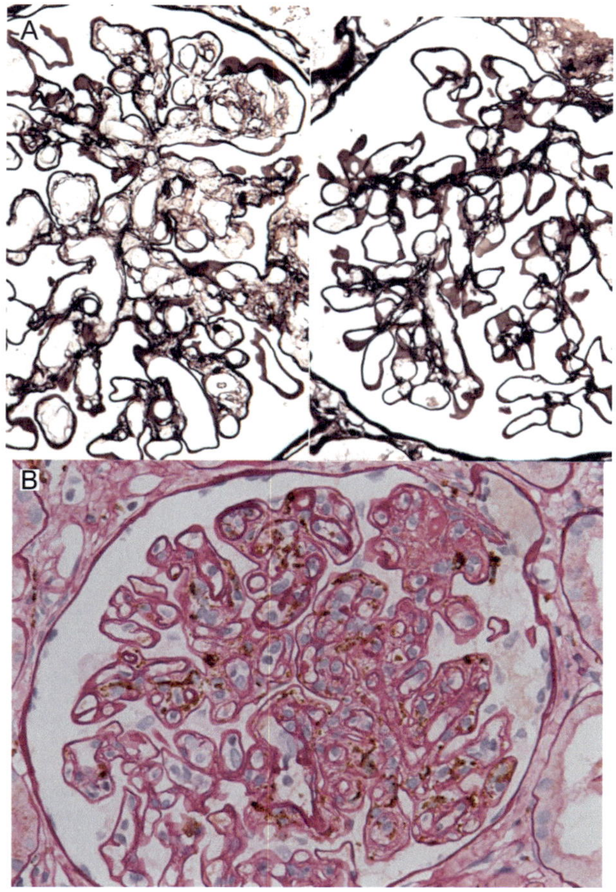

Figure 14.
Double contour formation in glomerulus with chronic glomerulitis in chronic active antibody mediated rejection-Banff score cg3 [(A) Jones, 400×] and normal glomerulus [(B) Jones, 400×]. Glomerulitis in chronic active antibody mediated rejection (Banff score g3, cg3) with diffuse double contour formation (glomerular capillaries with double contours are filled with swollen endothelial cells and inflammatory cells, among them macrophages predominate (CD68 and PAS, ×400).

3.2 Classification of antibody mediated rejection

According to Banff 2017 two types of ABMR were proposed-active ABMR (previously referred as acute ABMR) and chronic active ABMR [16].

The 2017 Banff meeting report noted the confusion generated by reports on acute and chronic ABMR, and emphasized the importance of correctly defining ABMR, including additional characteristics, like the nature of the antibody; the significance of C4d; the severity of microcapillary injury, gene transcripts, molecular and cellular signatures. As the previously used term acute ABMR was found to be misleading by the majority of the working group, the term active was elected to simply refer to lesions of ABMR with microvascular injury and evidence of current or recent antibody interaction with graft endothelium but without morphologic evidence of chronic vascular injury (transplant glomerulopathy, peritubular capillary basement membrane multilayering, new-onset arterial intimal fibrosis).

Two principal phenotypes defined in association of previously termed acute ABMR((1) ABMR phenotype 1 in the presensitized patient, occurring early post-transplant; and (2) ABMR phenotype 2, which develops from the emergence of

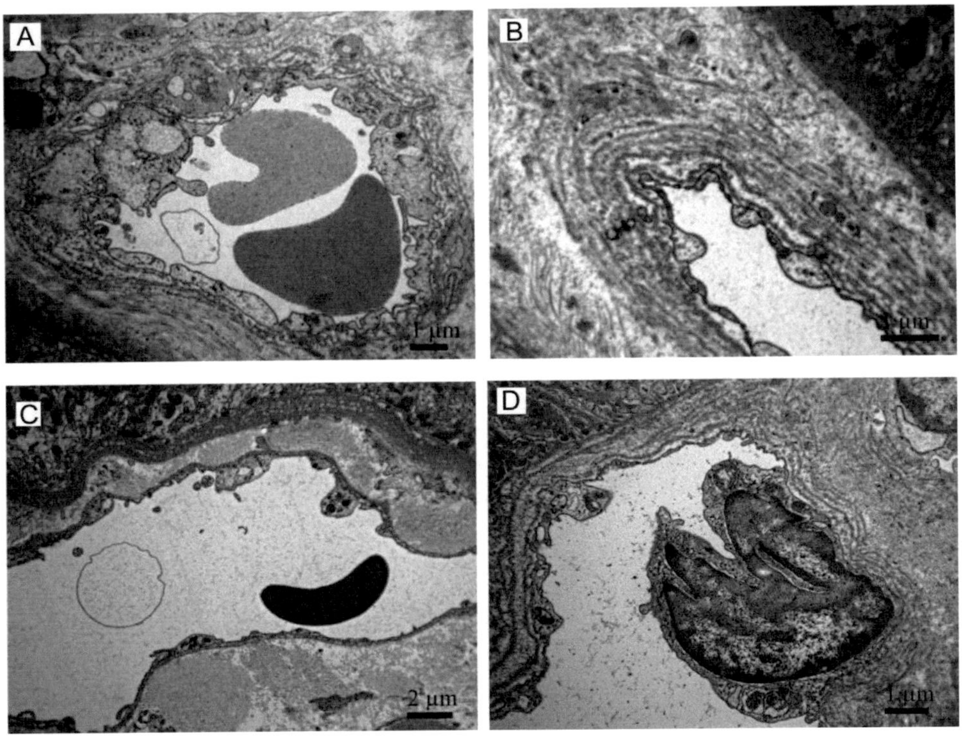

Figure 15.
Chronic active antibody mediated rejection: mild basement membrane multilamelation with swollen endothelium (A) and significant basement membrane multilamelation (B, D). Normal peritubular capillary (C, all electron micrographs).

According to revised Banff 2017 classification of antibody-mediated rejection (ABMR) in renal allografts *antibody-mediated changes* are classified in *Category 2, consisting of:*

Active ABMR; all 3 criteria must be met for diagnosis

1. Histologic evidence of acute tissue injury, including 1 or more of the following:
   - Microvascular inflammation (g > 0 and/or ptc > 0), in the absence of recurrent or de novo glomerulonephritis, although in the presence of acute TCMR, borderline infiltrate, or infection, ptc ≥ 1 alone is not sufficient and g must be ≥1
   - Intimal or transmural arteritis (v > 0)
   - Acute thrombotic microangiopathy, in the absence of any other cause
   - Acute tubular injury, in the absence of any other apparent cause
2. Evidence of current/recent antibody interaction with vascular endothelium, including 1 or more of the following:
   - Linear C4d staining in peritubular capillaries (C4d2 or C4d3 by IF on frozen sections, or C4d > 0 by IHC on paraffin sections)
   - At least moderate microvascular inflammation ([g + ptc] ≥2) in the absence of recurrent or de novo glomerulonephritis, although in the presence of acute TCMR, borderline infiltrate, or infection, ptc ≥ 2 alone is not sufficient and g must be ≥1
   - Increased expression of gene transcripts/classifiers in the biopsy tissue strongly associated with ABMR, if thoroughly validated
3. Serologic evidence of donor-specific antibodies (DSA to HLA or other antigens). C4d staining or expression of validated transcripts/classifiers as noted above in criterion 2 may substitute for DSA; however thorough DSA testing, including testing for non-HLA antibodies if HLA antibody testing is negative, is strongly advised whenever criteria 1 and 2 are met.

Chronic active ABMR; all 3 criteria must be met for diagnosis 4. Morphologic evidence of chronic tissue injury, including 1 or more of the following: • Transplant glomerulopathy (cg > 0) if no evidence of chronic TMA or chronic recurrent/de novo glomerulonephritis; includes changes evident by electron microscopy (EM) alone (cg1a) • Severe peritubular capillary basement membrane multilayering (requires EM) • Arterial intimal fibrosis of new onset, excluding other causes; leukocytes within the sclerotic intima favor chronic ABMR if there is no prior history of TCMR, but are not required 5. Identical to criterion 2 for active ABMR, above 6. Identical to criterion 3 for active ABMR, above, including strong recommendation for DSA testing whenever criteria 1 and 2 are met
C4d staining without evidence of rejection; all 4 features must be present for diagnosis 7. Linear C4d staining in peritubular capillaries (C4d2 or C4d3 by IF on frozen sections, or C4d > 0 by IHC on paraffin sections) 8. Criterion 1 for active or chronic, active ABMR not met 9. No molecular evidence for ABMR as in criterion 2 for active and chronic, active ABMR 10. No acute or chronic active TCMR, or borderline changes

Table 1.
Classification of antibody mediated rejection according to Banff 2017 [16].

de novo DSA in the late posttransplant period and is thought to be mostly related to nonadherence or inadequate immunosuppression) are not positioned in Banff 2017 classification.

In accordance with major advances in molecular biology and gene rearrangement, the diagnosis of ABMR is now dependent on histologic, serologic and transcriptomics findings (see **Table 1**) [16]. For detailed scoring explanations of histological lesions for antibody mediated rejection according to Banff 2017, please see **Table 2**.

Banff scoring for antibody mediated rejection	
v—vascular inflammation: the most severely affected artery dictates the score; an asterisk is added to the v score if interstitial hemorrhage or infarct present	v0: no arteritis v1: intimal arteritis with <25% luminal area lost (minimum = 1 cell, 1 artery) v2: intimal arteritis with ≥25% of luminal area lost in 1+ arteries v3: transmural arteritis or fibrinoid necrosis (medial smooth muscle necrosis) with lymphocyte infiltrate in vessels
g—glomerulitis: percentage of glomerular capillaries partially or completely occluded by inflammatory cells (polymorphonuclear leucocytes and mononuclear cells) and endothelial cell enlargement	g0: no glomerulitis g1: <25% of glomeruli involved (mostly segmental) g2: 25–75% of glomeruli involved (segmental to global) g3: >75% of glomeruli involved (mostly global)
ptc—peritubular capillaritis: the most severely affected peritubular capillary (PTC) dictates the score; an asterisk is added to the ptc score if neutrophils are lacking/only mononuclear cells are present	ptc0: <3 cells/PTC ptc1: 1+ inflammatory cells in >10% of cortical PTCs with 3–4 cells in most severely involved PTC ptc2: 1+ inflammatory cells in >10% of cortical PTCs with 5–10 cells in most severely involved PTC ptc3: 1+ inflammatory cells in >10% of cortical PTCs with >10 cells in most severely involved PTC

Banff scoring for antibody mediated rejection	
C4d—percentage of PTC (or vasa recta in the medulla) that has linear circumferential staining, scored in at least 5 high powered fields of cortex or medulla without scarring or infarct	C4d0: no staining of PTC and medullary vasa recta C4d1: <10% of PTC and medullary vasa recta C4d2: 10–50% of PTC and medullary vasa recta C4d3: >50% of PTC and medullary vasa recta
cg—transplant glomerulopathy: percentage of glomerular capillary loops with duplication of glomerular basement membrane in most affected nonsclerotic glomerulus	cg0: none by light microscopy (LM) and electron microscopy cg1a: only by electron microscopy in 3 glomerular capillaries cg1b: ≤25% by LM (1+ glomerular capillaries with glomerular basement membrane double contours by LM) cg2: 26–50% by LM cg3: >50% by LM
cv—transplant arteriopathy: arterial fibrointimal thickening; percentage of narrowing of lumen of most severely affected artery	cv0: none cv1: ≤25% of the luminal area cv2: 26–50% of the luminal area cv3: >50% of the luminal area

Table 2.
Detailed scoring explanations of histological lesions for antibody mediated rejection according to Banff 2017 [16].

3.3 Essential differences in comparison to previous classification

3.3.1 C4d in antibody mediated rejection

C4d is a split product of C4 activation and has no known biological action. It may be activated by the classical and lectin complement pathways. C4d staining is a specific marker of ABMR when the stain is deposited in the capillaries of kidney allograft and is now considered an alternative for DSA criterion in cases where DSA testing is not available or potentially false negative [17–19]. However, C4d staining has been shown to have significant limitations for diagnosis of ABMR due to low sensitivity, with negative results in up to 50% of patients with antibody-mediated rejection [4, 20]. Furthermore, C4d positivity has been reported in the absence of other evidence of graft injury as its expression depends on the density of PTCs and also may not be associated with measurable DSA in the case of non-HLA antibodies or antibodies absorbed by the allograft [21]. In studies comparing the risk of allograft loss among patients with consistently C4d negative ABMR vs. patients with C4d positive ABMR at a single center, both phenotypes were associated with statistically comparable increased graft loss compared with ABMR free matched controls. No clinical characteristics that reliably differentiated C4d negative and C4d positive ABMR were identified [22].

3.3.2 Expression of endothelium associated transcripts (ENDATs) in antibody mediated rejection

In patients with negative C4d staining, the diagnosis of ABMR may be confirmed on the basis of increased expression of gene transcripts or classifiers in the biopsy tissue that are strongly associated with ABMR [16].

Molecular markers associated with endothelial injury were first introduced into criteria of the ABMR classification in Banff 2013 [23]. Since that time, combinations of transcripts have been introduced and ABMR specific sets of transcripts proposed by different authors [16]. Data from Loupy et al. [4] showed that adding the results of the ABMR classifier to histologic findings significantly improved their ability to diagnose ABMR, independently from C4d and DSA.

However, it should be noted that at this point no specific Banff recommendations are given regarding which molecular transcript sets should be tested to assess gene expression. This includes the decision whether to perform molecular studies on freshly sampled tissue or FFPE. An advanced molecular approach using machine learning and classifiers has been done in recent years and has provided valuable information for improvement of rejection assessment [24]. The Alberta Transplant Applied Genomics Center team at the University of Alberta developed a "molecular microscope" approach to kidney transplant biopsies and has provided a system for distinguishing ABMR from other allograft pathologies by the expression of activated ENDATs. They proposed new rules to integrate molecular tests and histology into a precise diagnostic system that can reduce errors, ambiguity, and inter-pathologist disagreement [25].

4. Clinical features

In clinical setting ABMR can present as hyperacute (occurring within minutes after the vascular anastomosis), acute (occurring days to weeks after transplantation), late acute (occurring 3 months after transplantation), or chronic (occurring months to years after transplantation) [26–28].

4.1 Acute antibody mediated rejection

Acute ABMR almost always presents with an increase in serum creatinine, which is sometimes severe and accompanied with oligo-/anuria necessitating dialysis treatment. It is usually seen during the first few weeks after transplantation but can occur later, in which case it is usually associated with decreased immunosuppression or noncompliance [29]. The incidence varies with the amount of DSA present at the time of transplantation. In patients with high levels of DSA (i.e. sufficient to cause strongly positive crossmatch) the incidence may be as high as 40% in the first month after transplantation, while the incidence is less than 10% in patients with a negative crossmatch and DSA demonstrated only by solid phase assay [30, 31] According to Banff 2017 scoring system [16], histopathology in these patients is related to characteristics of *active ABMR*.

4.2 Chronic antibody mediated rejection

The diagnosis of chronic humoral rejection is usually, but not always, made in patients who are more than 6 months post transplantation [32]. The rise in serum creatinine is usually gradual and often accompanied by stepwise increase of proteinuria. Patients with chronic rejection are often hypertensive, sometimes nephrotic range proteinuria or even nephrotic syndrome can be observed. However, patients often have no clinical symptoms associated with chronic rejection, unless renal function is decreased enough that the patient has signs and symptoms of uremia. Except for proteinuria, urinalysis is usually unremarkable in chronic rejection. Contrary, in rare instances progression can be fairly rapid, especially with ongoing active lesions (chronic active ABMR), resulting in graft failure within months [33]. Chronic allograft injury is characteristically seen as transplant glomerulopathy on kidney biopsies. In addition to chronic features, signs of activity are often present, with prominent mononuclear cells in capillary loops with endothelial swelling (transplant glomerulitis) [34].

4.3 Subclinical antibody mediated rejection

A certain amount of kidney transplant recipients present with stable kidney graft function, but histological evidence of smoldering active ABMR on protocol biopsies [35]. These patients often have low-level DSAs (de novo or persistent/recurrent). Evidence suggests that untreated subclinical ABMR is an important predictor of poor renal allograft outcomes [36]. However, the lack of long-term follow-up data has prevented the development of strong guidelines for effective therapeutic interventions.

4.4 Hyperacute antibody mediated rejection

Nowadays, hyperacute rejection is a rare event in kidney transplantation affecting mostly presensitized patients (previous transplantation, blood transfusions, or pregnancy) [37]. It occurs due to preformed DSA present in high titers and presents as graft failure that can occur within minutes (but sometimes may be delayed for a few days) after transplantation [38]. The occurrence of this type of rejection is extremely rare, as preformed antibodies can usually be excluded by CDC crossmatch. However, there is growing evidence that there may exist hyperacute rejections mediated by endothelial, non-HLA antibodies that cannot be detected in standard T and B lymphocyte crossmatch techniques [39].

5. Treatment

Treatment for ABMR is not standardized, and there is still no evidence-based treatment guidelines. A recent therapy of ABMR in renal allografts is systematically reviewed by Wan et al. [2]. In addition to plasma exchange and intravenous immunoglobulin, which still present a backbone of treatment, a number of other therapies have been tried in small studies without consistent benefit, including anti-CD20, proteasome inhibitors, complement inhibitors, anti-interleukin-6 receptor blockers, and immunoglobulin G-degrading enzyme of *Streptococcus pyogenes* (IdeS).

5.1 IVIG

Intravenous immunoglobulin (IVIG) is used for treatment of ABMR, and it is used as an element of desensitizing protocols for ABO- and HLA-incompatible renal transplantation [40].

IVIG is prepared by human plasma from approximately 50,000–100,000 of healthy donors, composed of 90% intact IgG, a few dimers, Fabs (fragment antigen-binding) and traces of IgM and IgA [41].

There are many postulated immunomodulatory mechanisms of IVIG. Investigations in the early 1990s suggested the therapeutic potential of IVIG was due primarily to anti-idiotypic interactions with HLA antibodies [42]. Apart from its effects on B cells and phagocytes via Fc-gamma receptors, IVIG also functions as a scavenger of activated complement [43, 44].

Two general treatment protocols have been developed utilizing IVIG. The first is the use of high dose IVIG (2 g/kg) alone and the second is to combine lower dose IVIG with other modalities, usually plasmapheresis [45]. After the first successful report of Jordan et al. in 1998 [46] who treated acute ABMR in kidney and heart allografts by high-dose IVIG and methylprednisolone, there were more studies with usage of IVIG alone or in combination with plasmapheresis to show effectiveness in treatment of ABMR [47, 48].

Additional benefit of IVIG is its ability to replenish gamma globulin lost during therapeutic apheresis, decreasing infection risk [49].

5.2 Plasmapheresis

Both immunoabsorption (IA) and plasmapheresis (PP) are known to lower HLA-specific antibody levels in a variety of clinical settings [49]. Despite the substantial reductions in the titer of donor-specific anti-HLA antibodies achieved by IA and PP, the graft survival in these patients is significantly reduced, due to rebound synthesis of de novo alloantibodies.

PP is the most frequent modality applied and generally involves 1.0–1.5 volume exchange, using albumin as replacement. It is usually performed daily or every other day for an average of six sessions (up to 14 days). The initial treatment is typically a one-and-one-half-volume exchange with albumin, and subsequent treatments are a one-volume exchange with albumin. To avoid fresh frozen plasma administration, most clinicians prefer an every-other-day PP schedule as albumin alone can often be administered for replacement with interval recovery of the prothrombin time, partial thromboplastin time, and fibrinogen to acceptable levels. This avoids the risk of antigen sensitization. IA is a more selective modality that uses adsorbent membranes for antibody elimination [49, 50].

Few studies have been published where PP modalities are the sole or primary form of antibody reducing therapy [51–54]. However, PP alone has limited success in the treatment of ABMR, and this finding has led to the addition of therapies to prevent immunoglobulin resynthesis and B-cell proliferation. Therefore, PP is often used in combination with other antibody blocking (IVIG), suppression (rituximab, mycophenolate, calcineurin inhibitors), or depleting (bortezomib) modalities [2].

5.3 Rituximab and proteasome inhibitors

Rituximab is a chimeric monoclonal antibody directed against CD20, which is found on immature and mature B cells but not on plasma cells. Following treatment with rituximab, B cells undergo apoptosis and lysis [55]. Most adverse events are first infusion effects of generally mild severity. Additionally, an increased incidence of infections has been described including cases of progressive multifocal leukoencephalopathy [56], late onset Pneumocystis pneumonia [57] and fatal pneumococcus sepsis [58].

In renal transplantation rituximab is used for desensitization of highly sensitized patients or awaiting ABO-incompatible renal transplantation [59].

In case of ABMR, rituximab is used for the treatment of ABMR as a solo agent adjuncted to standard of care therapy [60, 61] or in some instances combined with bortezomib, a proteasome inhibitor causing apoptosis of mature plasma cells [62]. Treatment of ABMR with rituximab or bortezomib or combination in addition to standard therapy was in most instances partially effective on the short term, whereas treatment did not result in sufficient long-term graft survival [59–62].

The potential role of the anti-CD20 monoclonal antibody rituximab and the proteasome inhibitor bortezomib in decreasing the production of donor-specific anti-HLA antibodies and improving allograft survival in patients with antibody-mediated rejection was recently evaluated in two randomized, controlled trials RITUX ERAH [63] and BORTEJECT [64], but neither trial showed clinical benefits.

5.4 Complement inhibition

5.4.1 C5 inhibitors

Activation of the complement cascade in acute ABMR rejection has been identified as a major pathophysiological mechanism leading to allograft damage and dysfunction [65]. As a consequence, it has been proposed that specific inhibition of the recipient's complement system of limited duration may be useful to prevent acute ABMR.

The anti-C5 monoclonal antibody eculizumab, which inhibits terminal complement activation, was reported to decrease the incidence of early antibody-mediated rejection in HLA-sensitized renal-transplant recipients [66], although it failed to prevent chronic antibody-mediated rejection in recipients with persistently high levels of donor-specific anti-HLA antibodies [67]. It was also shown that preemptively usage of eculizumab following positive B-cell flow cytometric crossmatch transplant resulted in a reduced incidence of early ABMR from 41.0% in historical controls to 7.7% in eculizumab-treated patients [68].

5.4.2 C1 inhibitors

Binding of anti-HLA DSAs to complement fraction C1q, the first component in the activation of the complement cascade, has been associated with poor graft outcomes and severe phenotypes of ABMR [69]. These findings have provided the rationale for the use of proximal complement inhibition using C1 inhibitors (C1 INHs) in the treatment of ABMR. C1-INH is a serine protease inhibitor that inactivates both C1r and C1s and has multiple effects. Following antibody/immune complex activation of C1qrs, C1-INH dissociates C1r and C1s from the activated C1 macromolecule. This prevents proteolytic activation of C4 and C2 that form C3 convertase, which is important in the context of C4d deposition in AMR [70]. The use of a plasma-derived C1 INH in the treatment of active ABMR was evaluated in trial of 18 kidney transplant recipients with biopsy-proven, active ABMR [71], who were randomly assigned to receive C1 INH or placebo as adjunct therapy to standard-of-care treatment with PP, IVIG, and rituximab. Although there was no significant difference between the groups in posttreatment renal histopathology or graft survival on day 20, a trend toward sustained improvement in graft function at day 90 was observed in the C1 INH group.

Similar findings were reported in six kidney transplant recipients with active ABMR that were unresponsive to treatment with PP, IVIG, and rituximab [72]. All patients received the C1 INH Berinert (20 units/kg on days 1, 2, and 3 and then twice weekly) and high-dose IVIG (2 g/kg once per month) for 6 months. At 6 months, all patients showed an improvement in eGFR compared with baseline at the time of inclusion in the study. Renal allograft biopsies at 6 months revealed no significant change in histologic features; however, C4d deposition was observed in only one of six patients compared with five of six patients at baseline. In addition, of the six patients who were positive for a C1q-binding circulating DSA at the start of the study, only one had a positive DSA at 6 months.

5.5 IL-6 inhibition

The potential of proinflammatory cytokine blockade in kidney-transplant recipients with chronic ABMR has recently been highlighted [73]. Tocilizumab is a monoclonal antibody directed against the interleukin IL-6 receptor that has been used for the treatment of rheumatic diseases, such as rheumatoid arthritis and systemic juvenile idiopathic arthritis. Recently, tocilizumab was also evaluated as rescue therapy in 36 kidney transplant patients with chronic ABMR who failed standard-of-care treatment with IVIG and rituximab, with or without plasma exchange [74]. Tocilizumab was administered as 8 mg/kg monthly for 6 to 25 months. Significant reductions in DSAs and stabilization of renal allograft function were observed at 2 years. No significant adverse events or severe adverse events were reported.

5.6 IdeS

IgG-degrading enzyme of *Streptococcus pyogenes* (IdeS) cleaves at a very specific amino acid sequence in the hinge region of human IgG and essentially neutralizes all of the IgG in the body within 4 hours of administration. There is a period of about 7 days during which both soluble IgG and the B cell receptor are not detectable, after which it begins to rebound and can reconstitute fully by day 14 [75]. In clinical trials ideS was used in attempting to evaluate the efficacy to desensitize transplant patients with a positive crossmatch, where it showed efficacy in reduction of anti-HLA antibodies before kidney transplantation in patients who were HLA-incompatible with their donors [76, 77]. Further studies are necessary to evaluate IdeS treatment as a therapeutic strategy for ABMR.

5.7 Splenectomy

A desensitization protocol may be required to avoid ABMR in patients that are highly sensitized, have positive crossmatch or ABO incompatibility, however current protocols are not always effective to prevent ABMR and in some cases fail to convert subjects to a negative crossmatch before transplantation. Studies have shown that splenectomy can be successfully performed alone or in association with other treatments like bortezomib, rituximab or eculizumab to overcome severe ABMR, resistant to standard treatment [78–82].

In an effort to spare recipients the morbidity of a splenectomy, splenic irradiation in addition to other therapy may provide an effective intervention for rescuing and preserving allograft function [81].

6. Conclusions

Antibody-mediated rejection is an important cause of acute and chronic graft failure. Diagnosis of acute and chronic ABMR is based on typical histological hallmarks, positive C4d in peritubular capillaries and presence of donor-specific antibodies (DSA). Among standard of care treatment based on PP and IVIG, new treatment options have become available: B cell depletion (rituximab), plasma cell depletion (bortezomib), complement activation inhibition (c1 and c5 inhibitors), recently also IL-6 inhibitors and ideS. However, the high cost of novel medications and a lack of prospective studies evaluating their efficacy and safety limit the routine use of these agents in the treatment of ABMR in kidney transplant recipients.

Conflict of interest

Authors declare no conflicts of interest.

Author details

Nika Kojc[1] and Željka Večerić Haler[2]*

1 Institute of Pathology, Medical Faculty, University of Ljubljana, Ljubljana, Slovenia

2 Department of Nephrology, University Medical Centre Ljubljana, Ljubljana, Slovenia

*Address all correspondence to: zeljka.vecerichaler@kclj.si

References

[1] Sellares J et al. Understanding the causes of kidney transplant failure: The dominant role of antibody-mediated rejection and nonadherence. American Journal of Transplantation. 2012;**12**(2):388-399

[2] Wan SS et al. The treatment of antibody-mediated rejection in kidney transplantation: An updated systematic review and meta-analysis. Transplantation. 2018;**102**(4):557-568

[3] Morozumi K et al. Reviewing the pathogenesis of antibody-mediated rejection and renal graft pathology after kidney transplantation. Nephrology. 2016;**21**(Suppl 1):4-8

[4] Loupy A, Lefaucheur C. Antibody-mediated rejection of solid-organ allografts. The New England Journal of Medicine. 2018;**379**(12):1150-1160

[5] Kissmeyer-Nielsen F et al. Hyperacute rejection of kidney allografts, associated with pre-existing humoral antibodies against donor cells. Lancet. 1966;**2**(7465):662-665

[6] Adebiyi OO et al. Clinical significance of pretransplant donor-specific antibodies in the setting of negative cell-based flow cytometry crossmatching in kidney transplant recipients. American Journal of Transplantation. 2016;**16**(12):3458-3467

[7] McCaughan JA, Tinckam KJ. Donor specific HLA antibodies & allograft injury: Mechanisms, methods of detection, manifestations and management. Transplant International. 2018;**31**(10):1059-1070

[8] Hidalgo LG et al. De novo donor-specific antibody at the time of kidney transplant biopsy associates with microvascular pathology and late graft failure. American Journal of Transplantation. 2009;**9**(11):2532-2541

[9] Sypek M et al. HLA epitope matching in kidney transplantation: An overview for the general nephrologist. American Journal of Kidney Diseases. 2018;**71**(5):720-731

[10] Aubert O et al. Antibody-mediated rejection due to preexisting versus de novo donor-specific antibodies in kidney allograft recipients. Journal of the American Society of Nephrology. 2017;**28**(6):1912-1923

[11] Sapak M et al. Donor non-specific MICA antibodies in renal transplant recipients. Immunobiology. 2014;**219**(2):109-112

[12] Alvarez-Marquez A et al. Donor-specific antibodies against HLA, MICA, and GSTT1 in patients with allograft rejection and C4d deposition in renal biopsies. Transplantation. 2009;**87**(1):94-99

[13] Narayan S et al. Acute rejection associated with donor-specific anti-MICA antibody in a highly sensitized pediatric renal transplant recipient. Pediatric Transplantation. 2011;**15**(1):E1-E7

[14] Nickeleit V, Mengel M, Colvin RB. Renal transplant pathology. In: Jennete J, Olson J, Silva F, D'Agati V, editors. Heptinstall's Pathology of the Kidney. Philadelphia: Wolters Kluwer; 2015. pp. 1352-1379

[15] Stegall MD, Chedid MF, Cornell LD. The role of complement in antibody-mediated rejection in kidney transplantation. Nature Reviews. Nephrology. 2012;**8**(11):670-678

[16] Haas M et al. The Banff 2017 kidney meeting report: Revised diagnostic criteria for chronic

active T cell-mediated rejection, antibody-mediated rejection, and prospects for integrative endpoints for next-generation clinical trials. American Journal of Transplantation. 2018;**18**(2):293-307

[17] Correa RR et al. The importance of C4d in biopsies of kidney transplant recipients. Clinical & Developmental Immunology. 2013;**2013**:678180

[18] Haas M. C4d-negative antibody-mediated rejection in renal allografts: Evidence for its existence and effect on graft survival. Clinical Nephrology. 2011;**75**(4):271-278

[19] Sapir-Pichhadze R et al. A systematic review of the role of C4d in the diagnosis of acute antibody-mediated rejection. Kidney International. 2015;**87**(1):182-194

[20] Sis B et al. Endothelial gene expression in kidney transplants with alloantibody indicates antibody-mediated damage despite lack of C4d staining. American Journal of Transplantation. 2009;**9**(10):2312-2323

[21] Cohen D et al. Pros and cons for C4d as a biomarker. Kidney International. 2012;**81**(7):628-639

[22] Orandi BJ et al. Presentation and outcomes of C4d-negative antibody-mediated rejection after kidney transplantation. American Journal of Transplantation. 2016;**16**(1):213-220

[23] Haas M et al. Banff 2013 meeting report: Inclusion of c4d-negative antibody-mediated rejection and antibody-associated arterial lesions. American Journal of Transplantation. 2014;**14**(2):272-283

[24] Reeve J et al. Assessing rejection-related disease in kidney transplant biopsies based on archetypal analysis of molecular phenotypes. JCI Insight. 2017;**2**(12):pii: 94197. DOI: 10.1172/jci.insight.94197.eCollection 2017 Jun 15

[25] Halloran PF et al. Microarray diagnosis of antibody-mediated rejection in kidney transplant biopsies: An international prospective study (INTERCOM). American Journal of Transplantation. 2013;**13**(11):2865-2874

[26] Kim M et al. Antibody-mediated rejection in kidney transplantation: A review of pathophysiology, diagnosis, and treatment options. Pharmacotherapy. 2014;**34**(7):733-744

[27] Garg N et al. Defining the phenotype of antibody-mediated rejection in kidney transplantation: Advances in diagnosis of antibody injury. Transplantation Reviews. 2017;**31**(4):257-267

[28] Hasegawa J et al. Clinical and pathological features of plasma cell-rich acute rejection after kidney transplantation. Transplantation. 2018;**102**(5):853-859

[29] Nevins TE, Nickerson PW, Dew MA. Understanding medication nonadherence after kidney transplant. Journal of the American Society of Nephrology. 2017;**28**(8):2290-2301

[30] Gloor JM et al. Baseline donor-specific antibody levels and outcomes in positive crossmatch kidney transplantation. American Journal of Transplantation. 2010;**10**(3):582-589

[31] Schinstock C, Stegall MD. Acute antibody-mediated rejection in renal transplantation: Current clinical management. Current Transplantation Reports. 2014;**1**(2):78-85

[32] Baldwin WM 3rd, Valujskikh A, Fairchild RL. Mechanisms of antibody-mediated acute and chronic

rejection of kidney allografts. Current Opinion in Organ Transplantation. 2016;**21**(1):7-14

[33] Viglietti D et al. Dynamic prognostic score to predict kidney allograft survival in patients with antibody-mediated rejection. Journal of the American Society of Nephrology. 2018;**29**(2):606-619

[34] Katsuma A. Histopathological findings in transplanted kidneys. Renal Replacement Therapy. 2017;**3**(6). DOI: 10.1186/s41100-016-0089-0

[35] Yamamoto T et al. De novo anti-HLA DSA characteristics and subclinical antibody-mediated kidney allograft injury. Transplantation. 2016;**100**(10):2194-2202

[36] Loupy A et al. Outcome of subclinical antibody-mediated rejection in kidney transplant recipients with preformed donor-specific antibodies. American Journal of Transplantation. 2009;**9**(11):2561-2570

[37] Mengel M et al. Phenotypes of antibody-mediated rejection in organ transplants. Transplant International. 2012;**25**(6):611-622

[38] Zhang R. Donor-specific antibodies in kidney transplant recipients. Clinical Journal of the American Society of Nephrology. 2018;**13**(1):182-192

[39] Bharat A, Mohanakumar T. Immune responses to tissue-restricted nonmajor histocompatibility complex antigens in allograft rejection. Journal of Immunology Research. 2017;**2017**:6312514

[40] Montgomery RA et al. Desensitization in HLA-incompatible kidney recipients and survival. The New England Journal of Medicine. 2011;**365**(4):318-326

[41] Barahona A et al. The production processes and biological effects of intravenous immunoglobulin. Biomolecules. 2016;**6**(1):15

[42] Dietrich G, Kazatchkine MD. Normal immunoglobulin G (IgG) for therapeutic use (intravenous Ig) contain antiidiotypic specificities against an immunodominant, disease-associated, cross-reactive idiotype of human anti-thyroglobulin autoantibodies. The Journal of Clinical Investigation. 1990;**85**(3):620-625

[43] Spycher M et al. In vitro comparison of the complement-scavenging capacity of different intravenous immunoglobulin preparations. Vox Sanguinis. 2009;**97**(4):348-354

[44] Anthony RM et al. Intravenous gammaglobulin suppresses inflammation through a novel T(H)2 pathway. Nature. 2011;**475**(7354):110-113

[45] Jordan SC et al. Clinical aspects of intravenous immunoglobulin use in solid organ transplant recipients. American Journal of Transplantation. 2011;**11**(2):196-202

[46] Jordan SC et al. Posttransplant therapy using high-dose human immunoglobulin (intravenous gammaglobulin) to control acute humoral rejection in renal and cardiac allograft recipients and potential mechanism of action. Transplantation. 1998;**66**(6):800-805

[47] Tedla FM, Roche-Recinos A, Brar A. Intravenous immunoglobulin in kidney transplantation. Current Opinion in Organ Transplantation. 2015;**20**(6):630-637

[48] van Gent R, Metselaar HJ, Kwekkeboom J. Immunomodulation

by hyperimmunoglobulins after solid organ transplantation: Beyond prevention of viral infection. Transplantation Reviews. 2017;**31**(2):78-86

[49] Xie P et al. Plasmapheresis therapy in kidney transplant rejection. Blood Purification. 2019;**47**(1-3):73-84

[50] Clark WF et al. Plasmapheresis for the treatment of kidney diseases. Kidney International. 2016;**90**(5):974-984

[51] Madan AK et al. Treatment of antibody-mediated accelerated rejection using plasmapheresis. Journal of Clinical Apheresis. 2000;**15**(3):180-183

[52] Lennertz A et al. Plasmapheresis in C4d-positive acute humoral rejection following kidney transplantation: A review of 4 cases. Therapeutic Apheresis and Dialysis. 2003;**7**(6):529-535

[53] Allen NH et al. Plasma exchange in acute renal allograft rejection. A controlled trial. Transplantation. 1983;**35**(5):425-428

[54] Bohmig GA et al. Immunoadsorption in severe C4d-positive acute kidney allograft rejection: A randomized controlled trial. American Journal of Transplantation. 2007;**7**(1):117-121

[55] Pescovitz MD. Rituximab, an anti-cd20 monoclonal antibody: History and mechanism of action. American Journal of Transplantation. 2006;**6**(5 Pt 1):859-866

[56] Bohra C, Sokol L, Dalia S. Progressive multifocal leukoencephalopathy and monoclonal antibodies: A review. Cancer Control. 2017;**24**(4):1073274817729901

[57] Shelton E, Yong M, Cohney S. Late onset pneumocystis pneumonia in patients receiving rituximab for humoral renal transplant rejection. Nephrology. 2009;**14**(7):696-699

[58] Einecke G et al. Fatal pneumococcus sepsis after treatment of late antibody-mediated kidney graft rejection. Case Reports in Nephrology. 2018;**2018**:1415450

[59] Vo AA et al. Rituximab and intravenous immune globulin for desensitization during renal transplantation. The New England Journal of Medicine. 2008;**359**(3):242-251

[60] Waiser J et al. Comparison between bortezomib and rituximab in the treatment of antibody-mediated renal allograft rejection. Nephrology, Dialysis, Transplantation. 2012;**27**(3):1246-1251

[61] Moreso F et al. Treatment of chronic antibody mediated rejection with intravenous immunoglobulins and rituximab: A multicenter, prospective, randomized, double-blind clinical trial. American Journal of Transplantation. 2018;**18**(4):927-935

[62] Oblak T et al. Treatment of antibody-mediated rejection of kidney grafts with bortezomib and/or rituximab compared to standard regimen: Experience of Slovene National Center. Clinical Nephrology. 2017;**88**(13):91-96

[63] Sautenet B et al. One-year results of the effects of rituximab on acute antibody-mediated rejection in renal transplantation: RITUX ERAH, a multicenter double-blind randomized placebo-controlled trial. Transplantation. 2016;**100**(2):391-399

[64] Eskandary F et al. A randomized trial of bortezomib in late antibody-mediated kidney transplant rejection. Journal of the American Society of Nephrology. 2018;**29**(2):591-605

[65] Collins AB et al. Complement activation in acute humoral renal allograft rejection: Diagnostic significance of C4d deposits in peritubular capillaries. Journal of the American Society of Nephrology. 1999;**10**(10):2208-2214

[66] Tan EK et al. Use of eculizumab for active antibody-mediated rejection that occurs early post-kidney transplantation: A consecutive series of 15 cases. Transplantation. 2019. DOI: 10.1097/TP.0000000000002639. [Epub ahead of print]

[67] Kulkarni S et al. Eculizumab therapy for chronic antibody-mediated injury in kidney transplant recipients: A pilot randomized controlled trial. American Journal of Transplantation. 2017;**17**(3):682-691

[68] Stegall MD et al. Terminal complement inhibition decreases antibody-mediated rejection in sensitized renal transplant recipients. American Journal of Transplantation. 2011;**11**(11):2405-2413

[69] Bailly E et al. Prognostic value of the persistence of C1q-binding anti-HLA antibodies in acute antibody-mediated rejection in kidney transplantation. Transplantation. 2018;**102**(4):688-698

[70] Vo AA et al. A phase I/II placebo-controlled trial of C1-inhibitor for prevention of antibody-mediated rejection in HLA sensitized patients. Transplantation. 2015;**99**(2):299-308

[71] Montgomery RA et al. Plasma-derived C1 esterase inhibitor for acute antibody-mediated rejection following kidney transplantation: Results of a randomized double-blind placebo-controlled pilot study. American Journal of Transplantation. 2016;**16**(12):3468-3478

[72] Viglietti D et al. C1 inhibitor in acute antibody-mediated rejection nonresponsive to conventional therapy in kidney transplant recipients: A pilot study. American Journal of Transplantation. 2016;**16**(5):1596-1603

[73] Jordan SC et al. Interleukin-6, a cytokine critical to mediation of inflammation, autoimmunity and allograft rejection: Therapeutic implications of IL-6 receptor blockade. Transplantation. 2017;**101**(1):32-44

[74] Choi J et al. Assessment of tocilizumab (anti-interleukin-6 receptor monoclonal) as a potential treatment for chronic antibody-mediated rejection and transplant glomerulopathy in HLA-sensitized renal allograft recipients. American Journal of Transplantation. 2017;**17**(9):2381-2389

[75] Collin M, Bjorck L. Toward clinical use of the IgG specific enzymes IdeS and EndoS against antibody-mediated diseases. Methods in Molecular Biology. 2017;**1535**:339-351

[76] Jarnum S et al. The bacterial enzyme IdeS cleaves the IgG-type of B cell receptor (BCR), abolishes BCR-mediated cell signaling, and inhibits memory B cell activation. Journal of Immunology. 2015;**195**(12):5592-5601

[77] Jordan SC et al. IgG endopeptidase in highly sensitized patients undergoing transplantation. The New England Journal of Medicine. 2017;**377**(5):442-453

[78] Tzvetanov I et al. The role of splenectomy in the setting of refractory humoral rejection after kidney transplantation. Transplantation Proceedings. 2012;**44**(5):1254-1258

[79] Locke JE et al. The use of antibody to complement protein C5 for salvage treatment of severe antibody-mediated rejection. American Journal of Transplantation. 2009;**9**(1):231-235

[80] Orandi BJ et al. Eculizumab and splenectomy as salvage therapy for severe antibody-mediated rejection after HLA-incompatible kidney transplantation. Transplantation. 2014;**98**(8):857-863

[81] Orandi BJ et al. Splenic irradiation for the treatment of severe antibody-mediated rejection. American Journal of Transplantation. 2016;**16**(10):3041-3045

[82] Montgomery RA, Loupy A, Segev DL. Antibody-mediated rejection: New approaches in prevention and management. American Journal of Transplantation. 2018;**18**(Suppl 3):3-17

Section 3

Lung Transplantation: New Trends

Chapter 5

Perioperative Care for Lung Transplant Recipients: A Multidisciplinary Approach

Stacey H. Brann, Steven S. Geier, Olga Timofeeva, Norihisa Shigemura, Francis Cordova and Yoshiya Toyoda

Abstract

Lung transplantation has evolved as the gold standard for selective patients with end-stage lung disease since the first clinical lung transplant was performed in 1983 in the United States. Over the last few decades, lung transplantation volume has increased worldwide with steadily improving outcomes; however, access to lung transplantation remains limited due to the critical shortage of donor organs. Factors that have contributed to improved outcomes include a multidisciplinary management approach supported by advancements in surgical and anesthetic techniques, nursing and critical care, immunosuppressive therapy, transplant immunobiology, and the perioperative use of extracorporeal membrane oxygenation (ECMO) and ex vivo lung perfusion (EVLP). Excellent outcomes have been achieved in selective patients with high-risk comorbidities such as age over 65 years, concomitant severe coronary artery disease (CAD), and preexisting sensitization with donor-specific antibodies (DSAs). Such comorbidities are no longer considered absolute contraindications to lung transplantation. This chapter provides an overview of perioperative care of lung transplant recipients with focus on a multidisciplinary approach and highlights management strategies for patients with concomitant severe coronary artery disease and end-stage lung disease as well as those with preexisting sensitization with DSAs.

Keywords: perioperative care, lung transplantation, multidisciplinary management

1. Introduction

Lung transplantation has evolved as the gold standard for select patients with end-stage lung disease since the first clinical lung transplant was performed in 1983 in the United States. Over the last few decades, worldwide lung transplantation volume has steadily increased to approximately 4000 cases annually with progressive improvements in long-term survival. Perioperative management of lung transplant recipients is a highly complex endeavor. Crucial components include mechanical ventilation and weaning strategies, fluid management, and immunosuppression including induction therapy, management of rejection, perioperative antibiotics, antimicrobial prophylaxis, chest tube management, nutritional support, discharge planning, and education.

Optimal early outcomes are dependent on a well-coordinated, multidisciplinary approach. Factors that have contributed to improved outcomes include advancements in perioperative critical care, surgical and anesthetic techniques, improved immunosuppression and understanding of transplant immunobiology, stringent post-transplant surveillance for infection, rejection, and the perioperative use of extracorporeal membrane oxygenation (ECMO) [1] used to bridge decompensating patients to lung transplantation and ex vivo lung perfusion (EVLP) to facilitate optimization and transplantation of marginal donor lungs with outcomes considered equivalent to those from lungs transplanted using standard criteria [2, 3]. Given the aging population, older patients with a higher comorbid burden are being referred for lung transplant evaluation. In the United States, national registry data reveal a progressively increasing number of lung transplant recipients over age 70 years [4]. Advanced CAD is one such comorbidity that is no longer considered an absolute contraindication to lung transplantation. Excellent early outcomes have been reported with concomitant coronary artery bypass grafting (CABG) and lung transplantation [5]. However, the optimal treatment strategy for patients with concomitant advanced CAD and end-stage lung disease remains controversial, requires complex decision-making, and is evolving [6].

Highly sensitized transplant candidates, i.e., those with a high titer of preexisting HLA donor-specific antibodies (DSA), present unique challenges requiring specialized perioperative management. Antibody-mediated rejection (AMR) remains a problem without a reliable treatment in the care of lung transplant patients. AMR is usually mediated by anti-HLA DSA, and both pretransplant and posttransplant DSAs in lung transplant recipients are associated with acute rejection, chronic allograft dysfunction, and decreased survival [7, 8]. Patients transplanted with pretransplant DSAs are at a higher risk of hyperacute/accelerated acute ABMR, chronic rejection, and allograft loss across all solid organs [9]. Although several desensitization protocols have been reported for lung transplant candidates, the guidelines for protocol selection as well as criteria for successful response to treatment remain unclear [10–12].

In this chapter, an overview of general perioperative management of the lung transplant recipient is presented, including specific management strategies for concomitant advanced CAD and end-stage lung disease and perioperative management of the highly sensitized patient are presented.

2. A management algorithm for concomitant severe CAD in end-stage lung disease

As mentioned above, the optimal treatment strategy for high-risk patients with advanced CAD and end-stage lung disease remains controversial, requires complex decision-making, and is evolving. The author [SHB] presents an algorithm for management of these high-risk patients (**Figure 1**). Severe CAD is defined as an angiographically significant lesion (>70% stenosis) in at least one of the main coronary artery branches and/or when clinical or physiologic criteria demonstrate significant coronary flow limitation. An experienced interventional cardiologist and two cardiac surgeons jointly review the CAD severity of these patients upon referral for lung transplantation evaluation. Individualized treatment options are then formulated using the presented algorithm. For example, patients who become clinically unstable are hospitalized and urgently evaluated and are either listed for concomitant lung transplantation and CABG or CABG versus PCI, if deemed feasible, followed by lung transplantation depending on relative disease severity. If PCI prior to lung transplantation is deemed necessary, coronary lesion complexity and coronary stent characteristics determine the duration of dual antiplatelet therapy (DAPT) required to prevent in-stent restenosis. In general, more complex lesions require a longer duration of DAPT. Recommended DAPT duration by stent type is as follows: (i) Bare metal stent (ideal for patients anticipated to have a short wait list time)- one (1) month; (ii) Synergy stent- three (3) months; and (iii) typical second generation

DOI: http://dx.doi.org/10.5772/intechopen.85277

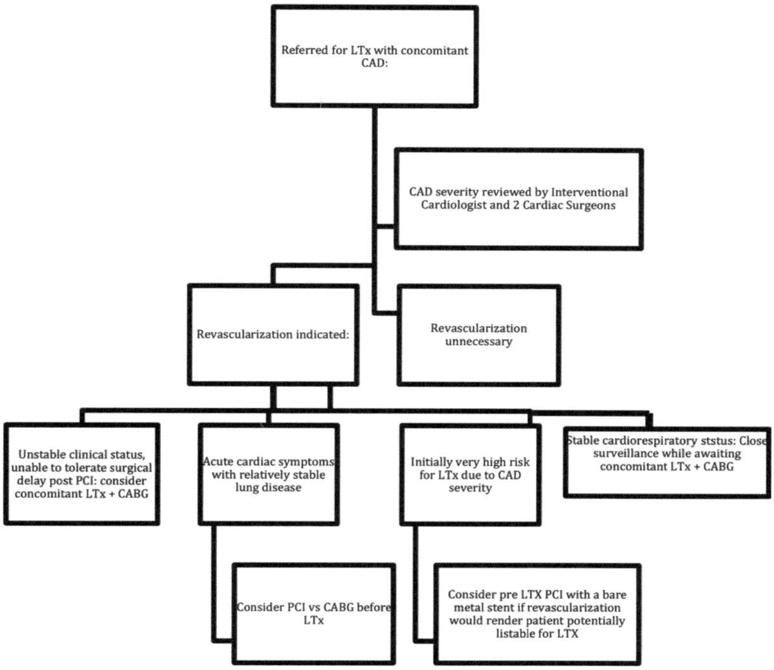

Figure 1.
Algorithm for management of patients with concomitant severe CAD and end-stage lung disease. LTX, lung transplant; PCI, percutaneous coronary intervention.

drug eluting stent- six (6) months. However, should lung transplantation become necessary before completion of DAPT, we proceed to lung transplantation albeit at a higher risk of perioperative bleeding. Close follow-up by the cardiologist and pulmonologist is maintained regardless of the treatment option.

3. Perioperative care of the lung transplant recipient

3.1 Intraoperative management

Preemptive management strategies that include meticulous and continuous cardiorespiratory monitoring, prompt initiation of vasoactive pharmacotherapy, volume administration, and institution of extracorporeal support are of critical importance during specific phases of intraoperative care. During these intraoperative phases of care (described below), there is a high risk of hemodynamic instability, lung derecruitment, worsening ventilation/perfusion mismatch, and alveolar hypoventilation leading to hypoxemia and hypercarbia in varying degrees of severity. The goals of perioperative ventilator support in lung transplantation rely on providing adequate minute ventilation while preventing oxygen toxicity, barotrauma, and volutrauma.

Specific problems that may occur during various intraoperative phases, and the recommended management strategies, are highlighted below:

3.1.1 Induction of anesthesia

Specific problems: acute RV decompensation due to (i) volume overload, (ii) decreased right ventricular (RV) preload and low cardiac output especially in the hypovolemic patient caused by increased intrathoracic pressure on commencement of positive pressure ventilation, (iii) Trendelenburg positioning, and (iv) medication-induced hypercarbia, hypoxia, and systemic hypotension leading to an acute exacerbation of preexisting pulmonary hypertension (PHTN) or severe new-onset PHTN.

Management strategies:

i. Invasive arterial blood pressure monitoring is required as hemodynamics can deteriorate rapidly in these patients.

ii. Temperature monitoring is mandatory as hypothermia exaggerates pulmonary vascular resistance (PVR) [13]. Core temperature can be measured with the pulmonary artery catheter.

iii. Following induction, orotracheal intubation options for selective lung ventilation include a double-lumen endotracheal tube or a single-lumen tube with a bronchial blocker, if a double-lumen tube cannot be passed successfully. The appropriate intubation strategy depends on laterality in cases of single-lung transplantation and surgical technique in particular whether the procedure will be performed using cardiopulmonary bypass (CPB) support. The intubation strategy should be discussed with the surgical team prior to induction.

iv. Initial ventilator parameters are adjusted according to the arterial blood gas (ABG) to maintain low arterial CO_2 tension and prevent hypoxemia. Suggested parameters include tidal volume 6–7 cc/kg body weight, a positive end-expiratory pressure (PEEP) of 5 cm H_2O, respiratory rate 14/min, inspired oxygen concentration (FiO_2) to maintain arterial oxygen saturation above 95%, and inspiration to expiration ratio (I:E) of 1:2 to prevent auto-PEEP especially in COPD patients.

v. Volume resuscitation is achieved with leukocyte-depleted packed red blood cells if the hemoglobin is <10 g/dL or colloid (albumin 5%) rather than crystalloid if the hemoglobin is >10 g/dL. Blood transfusion is minimized to due to the risk of allosensitization.

vi. Sedative agents should be administered with caution before induction as even minor respiratory depression may lead to increased PVR and acute RV decompensation.

vii. Pulmonary artery (PA) pressure monitoring via either a Swan-Ganz catheter or transesophageal echocardiography (TEE) is employed to guide anesthetic management, especially in high-risk patients.

viii. TEE monitoring is routinely performed (unless contraindicated) in all patients at the authors' institution to evaluate ventricular filling, ventricular function, and patent foramen ovale (PFO) status and to ensure correct Swan-Ganz catheter tip position in the main PA to prevent inadvertent catheter entrapment on clamping either branch PA. The probe is placed under the guidance of the attending anesthesiologist.

ix. Hemodynamic goals include avoidance of hypotension, bradycardia/tachycardia and exacerbation of PHTN. Heart rate and mean arterial pressure (MAP) goals are 60–100/min and 70–75 mmHg, respectively. An epinephrine infusion (2–4 μm/min) should be prepared and started in those patients with a preoperative history of, or evident, pulmonary hypertension or RV dysfunction. Baseline physiological assessment includes an ABG, a mixed venous blood gas (SvO_2) from the PA port of the Swan-Ganz catheter, and measurement of a thermodilution cardiac output.

x. Inhaled pulmonary vasodilator therapy, e.g., inhaled nitric oxide (INO) at 20 ppm, is used for all lung transplants at the authors' institution and is started following intubation.

xi. The surgical team as well as the perfusionist should be present in the room during anesthetic induction and be prepared to rapidly institute resuscitative measures that include emergent extracorporeal life support, such as peripheral veno-venous ECMO, veno-arterial ECMO, or CPB.

3.1.2 Preincision

Management strategies:

i. If the decision is made to use CPB or ECMO, a 70 mg/kg IV bolus of aminocaproic acid followed by an IV infusion at 30 mg/kg/h is given to minimize fibrinolysis.

ii. The induction immunotherapy protocols are detailed in Section 3.4.1 and Appendices (**Table 1**).

iii. Perioperative antibiotics: protocol details are provided in Section 3.5 below.

iv. For patients with a recent (<7 days) history of Coumadin administration, an IV infusion of vitamin K 10 mg diluted in 100 mL of normal saline is administered over 15 min.

Protocol for all patients except CMV mismatch, HBV/HCV/HIV infection, or history of malignancy
A. Induction (intraoperative): begin induction when final decision is made by the surgeons to accept the lungs
1. Premedication (30 min prior to alemtuzumab)
i. Methylprednisolone (Solu-Medrol): 1 g IV
ii. Acetaminophen (Tylenol): 650 mg PO/feeding tube
iii. Diphenhydramine (Benadryl): 50 mg IV
iv. Famotidine (Pepcid): 20 mg IV
2. Alemtuzumab (Campath) 30 mg IV over 2 h
3. Methylprednisolone (Solu-Medrol): additional dose of 250 mg IV prior to reperfusion of each lung
B. Postoperative Immunosuppression (Campath):
POD#1
1. Prednisone 5 mg orally or feeding tube daily; 10 mg if on chronic prednisone therapy preoperatively
2. Standard tacrolimus and mycophenolate mofetil/MMF (Cellcept) schedule

Table 1.
Induction therapy: Alemtuzumab (Campath).

3.1.3 Preimplantation

Management strategies:

i. An early trial of one-lung ventilation is advisable to see if acceptable gas exchange (pO_2, pCO_2, pH) and cardiac function can be maintained.

ii. To minimize a combustion hazard while using electrocautery:

- The FiO_2 should be minimized as tolerated during lung and bronchial dissection.
- On isolation of the lung for explantation, the appropriate lumen of the double-lumen endotracheal tube is suctioned with a flexible suction catheter to entrain room air when the bronchus is divided.

iii. If a vasoconstrictor infusion is needed to maintain blood pressure, options include vasopressin 0.01–0.04 units/min (institutional preference), norepinephrine 2–30 mcg/min, and phenylephrine 50–300 mcg/min, titrated to effect.

iv. Inotropic support may be provided either with IV infusions of epinephrine 2–10 mcg/min or milrinone 0.1–0.5 mcg/kg/min (renally dosed as appropriate), titrated to achieve a normal cardiac output and index.

v. Immediately prior to reperfusion of each transplanted lung, the surgeon will request an additional bolus of methylprednisolone 250 mg IV.

vi. In preparation for reperfusion, the hemodynamic status should be optimized in anticipation of volume loss to the transplanted organ and peripheral vasodilation resulting from washout of vasoactive substances when the allograft is unclamped.

3.1.4 Postimplantation to lung allograft reperfusion/reexpansion

Specific problems: systemic vasodilatation and hypotension, reperfusion pulmonary edema (increased vascular permeability and loss of lymphatic drainage), and hyperacute rejection.

Management strategies:

i. On completion of the vascular anastomoses, a controlled reperfusion maneuver is performed by gradually releasing the pulmonary artery clamp to prevent the development of allograft reperfusion pulmonary edema.

ii. Initial re-expansion of the donor lung is achieved with a sustained Valsalva maneuver to 30 cm H_2O, and interruptions to ventilation should be minimized thereafter.

iii. The ventilation strategy immediately posttransplant is intended to minimize injury to the donor lung from either mechanical factors or oxygen free radicals: typical settings will be FiO_2 0.40, PEEP 10 cm H_2O, rate 20/min, and TV 6 mL/kg (donor weight).

iv. Peripheral pulse oximeters are frequently inaccurate around the time of reperfusion, and the SvO_2 may be used as an indirect measure of adequate oxygen exchange.

v. If oxygenation is inadequate, FiO_2 may be increased in a stepwise fashion up to 0.60 while communicating these changes with the surgeon.

vi. If graft performance is initially inadequate, consideration should be given to temporarily support gas exchange with ECMO rather than use a sustained high FiO_2.

vii. Five minutes after reperfusion, an ABG should be checked.

viii. After reperfusion, the TEE should be used to assess for LV and RV function, the presence of air in the left heart, and evidence of stenosis at the pulmonary vein anastomoses.

ix. A thermodilution cardiac output should be measured and recorded following reperfusion and after chest closure.

x. A cardiac index of 2.2–2.5 is ideal—higher rates of pulmonary blood flow may increase the risk of significant pulmonary edema. Specific hemodynamic optimization strategies are detailed in Section 3.1.3 above.

xi. Because of the adverse effects on donor lung function, the requirement for blood products should be agreed upon between the attending anesthesiologist and surgeon.

xii. The double-lumen ETT tube will need to be changed to a single-lumen ETT at the end of the case to facilitate flexible bronchoscopy for anastomosis surveillance and tracheobronchial toilet. The FiO_2 should be increased transiently to 1.0 before this procedure.

3.1.5 Chest closure

Specific problems: restrictive chest cavity dynamics caused by:

i. Direct lung allograft compression leading to acute allograft dysfunction manifested by decreased compliance, derecruitment, and ventilation-perfusion mismatch. Etiologies include excessive donor-recipient size mismatching, noncompliant "frozen" pleural cavity associated with pulmonary fibrosis, severe pleural thickening and/or calcification, asymmetric chest cavities, severe kyphoscoliosis, and diaphragmatic elevation.

ii. Direct cardiac compression resulting in a cardiac tamponade physiology.

Management strategies include:

- Immediately reopening the chest
- Ventilator adjustments to prevent barotrauma, i.e., transient reductions in TV and/or PEEP
- Volume administration to optimize preload
- Leaving the intercostal space open with closure of only the muscular, subcutaneous tissue and skin layers or lung volume reduction followed by attempted reclosure.

3.1.6 Disruption to positive pressure ventilation

This can occur during (i) ventilator disconnection prior to patient bed to bed transfer, (ii) switching to a single-lumen endotracheal tube to facilitate postprocedure bronchoscopy, (iii) airway dislodgement, and (iv) manual ventilation while the patient is being transported. Gentle Valsalva maneuvers to 30 cm H_2O are performed immediately after any disruptions to positive pressure ventilation.

3.1.7 The use of pulmonary vasodilator therapy

The use of pulmonary vasodilator therapy with INO or epoprostenol (Flolan) is indicated for: (i) hypoxemia during single-lung ventilation, (ii) refractory hypoxemia in severe primary graft dysfunction (PGD), (iii) to prevent/mitigate exacerbations in PHTN and subsequent cardiorespiratory perturbations during induction and pulmonary artery clamping and thus potentially avoiding the institution of CPB [14].

3.2 Intensive care unit management

Initial postoperative care for all lung transplant recipients is provided on the intensive care unit. Interventions specific to the care of the lung transplant patient will include, but are not limited to, the following:

i. *Ventilator management*: The goal is to provide adequate minute ventilation while preventing oxygen toxicity, barotrauma, and volutrauma. As such, ventilatory parameters are individualized and adjusted to achieve these goals. The aim is early extubation as soon as is clinically feasible. Recommended ventilatory parameters are detailed in Section 3.1.4 above. In particular, the goal is the use the lowest FiO_2 to maintain arterial oxygen saturations greater than 91% and a tidal volume based on donor height (where possible) to prevent/minimize PGD [15, 16].

ii. *INO weaning protocol*: In single-lung transplants for pulmonary fibrosis, the author [SB] recommends weaning INO first (if used) within the first 6–12 h followed by oxygen and PEEP weaning, as tolerated. In single-lung transplants for COPD, the PEEP is weaned first (to prevent compression of the less compliant lung allograft by the hyperinflated native lung) followed by INO (within 6–12 h) and oxygen weaning, as tolerated. After double-lung transplants, the goal is to wean INO within 24 h. Following extubation, the patient will be instructed in the use of the incentive spirometer and the flutter valve. Early mobilization out of bed to chair is instituted.

iii. *Hemodynamic management and fluid administration protocol*: Due to the propensity of lung allografts to develop pulmonary edema (altered tissue hydrostatic forces, endothelial dysfunction, destruction of lymphatic drainage channels), the goals are to maintain adequate cardiac output; avoid high cardiac output states; wean inotropes rapidly when no longer clinically indicated; use colloid (albumin 5%) rather than crystalloid for volume replacement; medication infusions are concentrated to reduce volume loading; maintain hemoglobin at 10 g/dL with leukocyte-depleted packed red blood cells, CVP 10–12 mmHg, and MAP 65–75 mmHg; and adjust appropriately for urine output above 0.5 mL/kg body weight, $SvO_2 > 65\%$, and lactate <2 mmol/L. Additional blood products are given per clinical need (FFP, cryoprecipitate, and platelets).

- A cardiac index of 2.2–2.5 is ideal—to minimize the risk of significant pulmonary edema. Specific hemodynamic optimization strategies are detailed in Section 3.1.3 above. Serial lactate levels and SvO_2 are measured every 6 h or as needed depending on clinical status.

- Once clinically stable and not on high-dose pressors, aggressive diuresis as dictated by the patient's clinical status and radiographic findings is initiated with Lasix 20–40 mg IV every 8 h or a Lasix infusion 0.5–4 mg/min, titrated to achieve a negative intake/output balance (500 mL to 1 L) over the initial 24 h.

iv. Postoperative pain and sedation management: Important goals include use of the lowest effective dose and timely weaning of opioids such as fentanyl infusion 0.5–1.5 mcg/kg/h or 50–100 mcg IV boluses every 1–2 h (use renal dosing where applicable), sedatives such as Precedex 0.2–1.4 mcg/kg/h, and anxiolytics such as Versed 0.02–0.1 mg/kg/h to prevent respiratory depression, hypotension, oversedation, and delayed extubation.

v. *Flexible bronchoscopy* is performed on all patients prior to extubation to facilitate tracheobronchial toilet and to evaluate the integrity of the airways.

vi. *Chest tube removal* is started in POD#1 once criteria are met (no air leak, total serosanguineous drainage <200 mL/24 h, and/or <20 mL/h for the three consecutive hours prior to planned removal). Our institutional protocol involves removal of the posterior-dependent chest tube first, conversion of the anterior and middle chest tubes to H_2O seal, and removal of the anterior and last the middle chest tube when the patient has been ambulant to minimize residual pleural effusion collections.

vii. *Nutritional support*: While oral intake of all medications and nutrition is preferred, the patient will undergo a swallowing assessment 24–48 h following extubation and a nutritional assessment within 48 h after admission to the ICU. Until oral intake is established, for patients deemed at high risk of aspiration, a postpyloric naso-enteric feeding tube is placed immediately on extubation. In low-risk patients, orogastric tube feeds are started shortly after arrival to the ICU absent contraindications that include known severe gastroesophageal reflux disease, gastric distension, esophageal dysmotility syndromes, and high pressor requirements. The dietitian will make individualized recommendations for the patient's nutritional needs and will follow the patient throughout the hospitalization and make recommendations to the team accordingly. Gastroenterology consultation will be initiated as warranted by the patient's condition.

viii. *DVT prophylaxis* will be initiated per hospital protocol (subcutaneous heparin 5000 units every 8 h). Weekly surveillance upper and lower extremity Doppler studies are performed.

ix. *Physical therapy consultation* will be completed within 48 h of transplantation; early mobility is the goal.

3.2.1 Primary graft dysfunction

PGD is an acute manifestation of ischemia-reperfusion injury associated with multiple risk factors (donor-derived and related to procurement/preservation and reperfusion) with a peak incidence within the first 72 h after lung transplantation [17, 18]. The severity of PGD is graded based on the presence or absence of diffuse opacities on chest radiograph and the ratio of arterial oxygen pressure to inspired oxygen concentration, i.e., the PaO_2/FiO_2 ratio. The severity ranges from grade 0 (absent radiographic infiltrates, any PaO_2/FiO_2 ratio, extubated patient with/without supplemental oxygen) to grade 3 (radiographic infiltrates present bilaterally or, if single-lung transplant—absent in the native lung, PaO_2/FiO_2 ratio <200, mechanical ventilation with FiO_2 >50% for 48 h, requirement for extracorporeal life support). Severe PGD negatively impacts short-term outcome after lung transplantation (30-day mortality up to 50%) and is also associated with the development of chronic allograft dysfunction, i.e., bronchiolitis obliterans syndrome [15, 19, 20]. Management of PGD is predominantly supportive, i.e., cardiorespiratory support including lung protective ventilation, inhaled pulmonary vasodilator therapy, fluid and transfusion restriction, diuretic therapy, and extracorporeal life support for refractory hypoxemia with/without hemodynamic instability [21, 22].

3.2.2 The role of extracorporeal support: ECMO versus CPB in lung transplantation

In the United States, the rate of CPB use during lung transplantation varies widely. CPB provides hemodynamic stability with the heart in a decompressed state, which affords technical advantages by reducing right heart distension and vascular wall tension/shear stress, especially in the presence of moderate pulmonary hypertension. This facilitates nontraumatic vascular clamping and the performance of tension-free anastomoses. However, several studies have reported worse early postoperative outcomes as compared to off-pump lung transplantation [23, 24]. ECMO as an alternative to CPB provides certain advantages: reduced heparin requirements, reduced systemic inflammatory response, and coagulopathy resulting in less bleeding and lower transfusion requirements. Additionally, ECMO can be continued into the early postoperative period to facilitate allograft recovery while optimizing cardiorespiratory support.

3.3 Immunologic assessment of the lung transplant recipient

To decrease the immunologic AMR risk posttransplant, high-titer pretransplant DSAs that result in positive complement-dependent cytotoxicity (CDC) crossmatch and cause hyperacute rejection should be effectively avoided or preemptively treated based on acceptable risk defined by the transplant center. However, antibody avoidance results in longer waiting times and death on waiting list. At TUH, about 13% of waitlisted patients have CPRA > 80% (11 out of 83 active patients), but only about 3.5% of transplanted patients have CPRA > 80% (12 out of 345 patients transplanted between 2016 and 2017), showing a disparity in transplantation rates for highly sensitized patients (**Figure 2**). In thoracic transplantation, the use of the virtual crossmatch without a prospective serologic crossmatch became the standard practice. In virtual crossmatch, compatibility between donor and recipient is predicted by comparing the recipient's HLA-specific antibodies with the HLA antigens of the prospective donor. The primary method for antibody identification is the solid-phase single-antigen bead (SAB) assay that provides information about antibody specificities and their relative strengths based on mean fluorescence intensity (MFI) readout. **Figure 3** shows examples of positive and negative virtual crossmatches performed using SAB results that allow evaluation of compatibility between the donor and the recipient. However, there are several limitations to accurate virtual crossmatching based on SAB assay alone, including (1) that SAB assay is prone to detection of the so-called naturally occurring antibodies against denatured/cryptic antigens and that (2) it is not clearly understood at what MFI threshold DSA should be considered as clinically relevant [25].

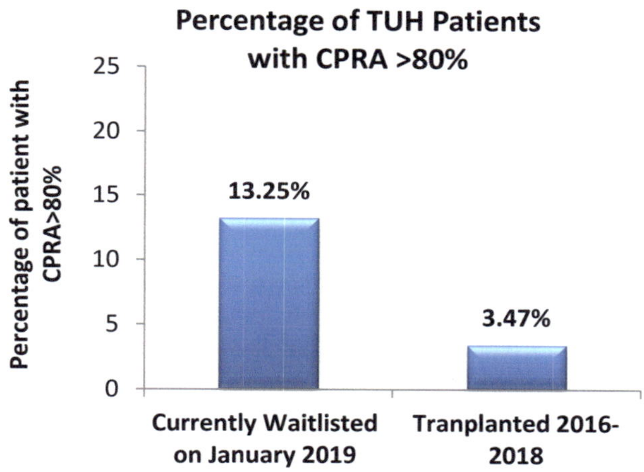

Figure 2.
Only 4% of transplanted patients (12/296) have CPRA > 80%, while 13% (11/83) patients on the waitlist have CPRA >80%.

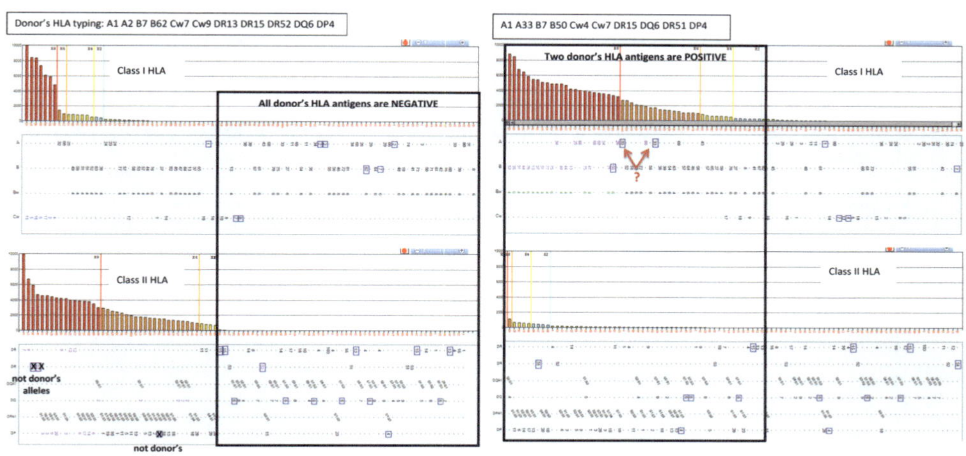

Figure 3.
Examples of negative (A) and positive (B) virtual crossmatches using results of single-antigen bead assay.

The precise role of naturally occurring antibodies is not well understood yet, but several studies suggest that such antibodies do not have clinical significance [26–29]. Usually antibodies against cryptic epitope do not result in positive flow cytometric or CDC crossmatches and do not impact clinical posttransplant outcomes. Several reports demonstrated that some antibodies detected in SAB assays may be directed against cryptic epitopes on recombinant HLA proteins created by missing peptides and/or b2-macroglobulin [30]. Other studies estimate that about 20–30% of waitlisted patients have antibodies against denatured antigens [28]. The naturally occurring antibodies can easily be recognized by negative reactions in cell-based crossmatch testing, but thoracic programs rarely have a luxury of performing a prospective crossmatch. Therefore, when/if not recognized as antibodies against denatured antigens, these specificities can deny an organ transplant based on virtual crossmatch. Starting in October 2016, our center began modifying our existing HLA testing protocols to better identify patients with and without pretransplant DSA by using multiple assay platforms, including FlowPRA Screen, phenotypic beads, and the well-established single-antigen beads. We studied 58 consecutive

VXM performed during July–December 2016 for lung candidates with CPRA>10%. Twenty-eight patients had no DSAs or had acceptably weak DSAs; they proceeded to transplant based VXM. All retrospective flow crossmatches were negative. The other 30 patients had positive VXM due to one or more moderate to strong DSAs, and the organ offers were refused. We found that 7 out of 30 (23.3%) VXM were called unacceptably positive due to the presence of antibody against denatured antigens [31]. Among these seven patients, three patients had antibodies against class I denatured antigens (2500–3500 MFI), and four patients had antibodies against class II denatured antigens (2000–14,000 MFI). We also found that by using LSPRA (Phenotypic Bead) and FlowPRA Screen assays along with SAB, we can preemptively recognize antibodies against denatured antigens not to deny organ offers unnecessarily. Instead of performing VXM using only SAB results, we now confirm that donor's antigens are positive by other assays as well (**Figure 3A**). Whenever antibody is detected only by SAB assay, it is considered to be directed against a cryptic epitope and, therefore, to be clinically irrelevant and not able to cause positive flow cytometry crossmatch (**Figure 4A**). DSAs detected by both SAB and phenotypic bead assays are considered as antibody against native HLA antigens (**Figure 4B**). The "true" DSAs undergo evaluation for strength as described below. Using this strategy we successfully transplanted five out of seven patients who were denied offers during July–December 2016 period. Since January 2017, all transplant candidates undergo antibody testing by SAB and LSPRA/FlowPRA Screen assays, so the presence of antibodies against cryptic epitopes can be easily recognized at the time of donor evaluation. This strategy results in reducing the number of unacceptable antigens and reduces percentage

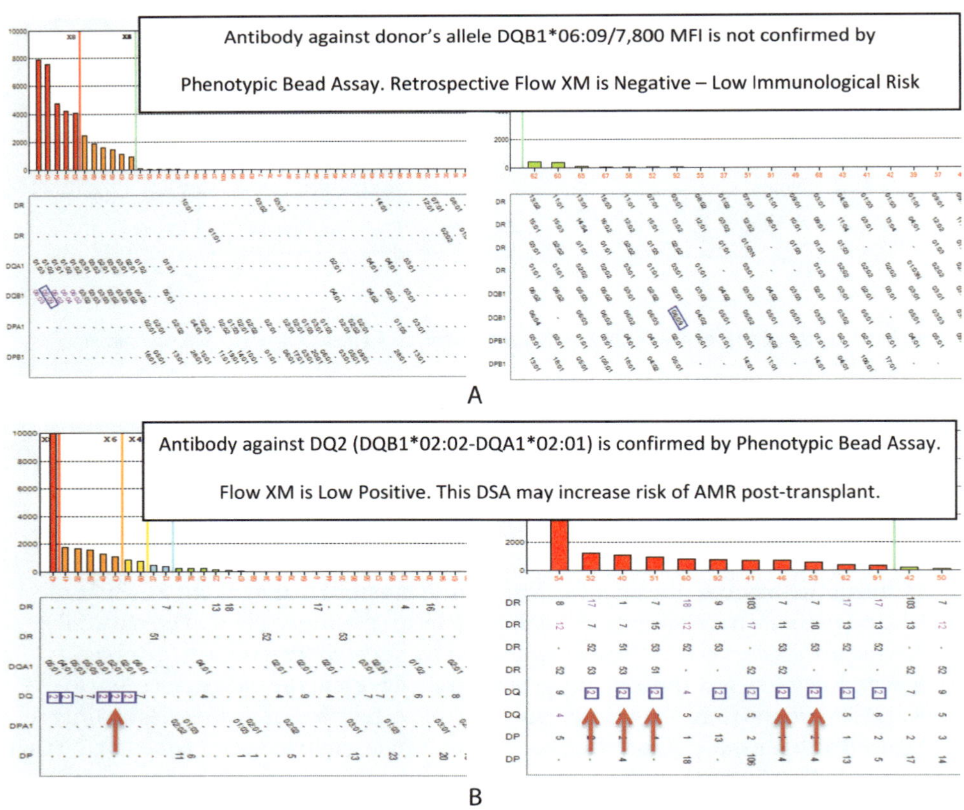

Figure 4.
Accuracy of virtual crossmatch can be improved by performing SAB alone with screening assays.

of CPRA (the percent of incompatible donors). Our data on relevance of antibodies against cryptic epitopes correlate well with several recent studies, including meta-analysis of 13 cohorts of lung recipients (total 3039 patients) showed that only DSAs that were detected by both SAB and screening assays were associated with CLAD (HR = 2.02, 95% CI = 1.37–2.97, P < 0.001). When DSAs were detected by SAB alone, the association with CLAD was no longer significant [32]. Overall, our experience is that use of SAB assay by itself may unnecessarily deny an organ offer due to the false-positive reactions and that use of screening assays improves the accuracy of virtual crossmatches and provides additional opportunities for sensitized patients.

Another important consideration is how to determine a threshold level below which DSA is clinically irrelevant or manageable perioperatively. Mean fluorescence intensity units somewhat indicate the quantity of antibody binding, when serum is pretreated with EDTA to inactivate complement and remove prozone-like inhibition in SAB assay. It is important to note that when untreated serum is used, the correlation between MFI and antibody quantity is very poor [33]. MFI values cannot be reliably measured above 20,000 MFI due to saturation effect, and intercenter studies suggest that the positive cutoff for DSA should be ~1500 MFI [33]. At TUH, antibodies <3000 are considered as weak and can be crossed without perioperative treatment, while antibodies >10,000 strong in general considered as strong and present unacceptably high risk. For patients with CPRA < 50%, UA are listed in UNET based on 3000 MFI cutoff. However, for patients with CPRA >50%, the immunologic management strategy differs depending on the urgency for transplant and the strength of antibody specificities.

Data from our center show that it is possible to reduce HLA antibody levels temporarily using various protocols, including high dose of IVIG plus Rituxan or five plasma exchanges with or without bortezomib (Velcade) followed by high dose of IVIG. However, if not transplanted during that "window of opportunity," the patient's antibodies invariably rebound and sometimes to the levels even higher than prior to initiation of desensitization. Even for patients with high LAS, who receive a priority during allocation, it is not easy to predict when a "compatible" donor may become available. Instead of implementing desensitization while patients are waiting for the offers, the Toronto Lung Transplant Program has developed a perioperative desensitization protocol-guiding organ allocation and maintenance immunotherapy [34]. At TUH, Toronto's protocol is implemented with some modifications. Highly sensitized patients with antibodies >3000 MFI are additionally tested at 1:16 serum dilution. Antibodies that become <3000 MFI at 1:16 are usually not listed as unacceptable antigens (UA) in UNET, while antibodies >3000 MFI at 1:16 are generally listed as UA. Our center experience is that antibodies <3000 MFI would result in borderline or low-positive flow cytometry crossmatch and can be managed postoperatively as needed. Therefore, if antibody decreases to <3000 at 1:16 dilution, it will result only at most in low-positive flow crossmatch after a single plasma exchange. This additional step allows us to avoid a prospective crossmatch for rapidly declining patients with high CPRA and to accept an offer based on VXM. The treatment usually continues posttransplant with additional 4–5 plasma-exchange sessions, followed by high dose of IVIG and Rituxan as needed. The perioperative desensitization is implemented at the time of transplant decision-making, which reduces unnecessary treatments and the risk of complications for patients who did not proceed to transplant.

3.4 Immunosuppressive therapy

3.4.1 Induction therapy

Induction therapy is determined at the time of listing and is modified for the patient as medically indicated. Induction therapy is administered in the operating room by the anesthesiologist. Exceptions to the standard therapy are documented in the patient's medical record. Alemtuzumab (Campath) is the first-line induction therapy (**Table 1**). Basiliximab (Simulect) is given to patients with cytomegalovirus (CMV) mismatch, Hepatitis B virus (HBV)/HCV/HIV infection, and/or a history of malignancy (**Table 2**).

3.4.2 Postoperative immunosuppression

i. Postoperative immunosuppression is a combination therapy including a calcineurin-inhibitor therapy (CIT), steroids, and antimetabolite therapy. The postoperative immunosuppression administration and dosing guidelines are found in **Tables 1–3**.

ii. Tacrolimus is the first-line CIT and is initiated on the first postoperative day (POD) #1 via the sublingual route of administration. Initiation of tacrolimus may be held at the discretion of the lung transplant surgeon and/or transplant pulmonologist if the patient is not hemodynamically stable, aggressive diuresis is required, or there is evidence of renal complications. Oral medication will be administered when the patient has been cleared for oral intake. The intravenous route of administration is not preferred.

iii. Postoperative steroid therapy begins on POD #1 and the dosing is based on the specified induction therapy for the patient.

iv. Mycophenolate mofetil (Cellcept) is the first-line antimetabolite and begins on POD #1 if the platelet count is greater than 40,000 and rising and the lymphocyte count is greater than 10. The dose is reevaluated daily for titration to goal of 750 mg Q12 h.

v. For patients receiving basiliximab (Simulect) based induction, an additional dose of basiliximab (Simulect) is administered on POD #4.

Protocol for patients with CMV mismatch HBV/HCV/HIV infection, or history of malignancy		
A. Induction (intraoperative): begin induction when final decision is made by the surgeons to accept the lungs 1. Basiliximab (Simulect) 20 mg IV and methylprednisolone (Solu-Medrol) 1 g IV at the start of the procedure 2. Methylprednisolone (Solu-Medrol): additional dose of 250 mg IV prior to reperfusion of each lung		
B. Postoperative immunosuppression (Simulect)		
1. POD #1 Steroid taper		
Begin with methylprednisolone (Solu-Medrol) IV and switch to prednisone when tolerating PO		
POD	Prednisone (mg)	Methylprednisolone (mg)
1	50 daily	20 Q 12 h
2	40 daily	32 daily
3	30 daily	24 daily
4–14	20 daily	16 daily
15	15 daily	12 daily Taper dose to 0.1 mg/kg/day by 3 months
2. Standard tacrolimus (Prograf) and MMF (Cellcept) schedule		
POD #4 Basiliximab (Simulect) 20 mg IV		

Table 2.
Induction therapy: Basiliximab (Simulect).

POD#1 1. Tacrolimus (Prograf) 0.5 mg orally or sublingual Q 12 h (target 10–12): IV route is to be avoided. Begin when patient is hemodynamically stable and aggressive diuresis is not required. For split doses, the higher dose is scheduled for the evening
2. MMF (Cellcept) 250 mg orally or feeding tube Q 12 h: dose if lymphocyte count greater than or equal to 10 and/or platelet count greater than or equal to 40 K (oral dose = IV dose). Reevaluate daily for titration to goal of 750 mg Q 12 h
Prograf dose on the day of discharge from initial transplant admission is required to be greater than or equal to 6

Table 3.
Postoperative immunosuppression: all patients.

3.4.3 Maintenance and monitoring of immunosuppressant levels

Daily tacrolimus level measurements are taken. The target tacrolimus level is 10–15 ng/dl with a goal level of 12. In general, once the tacrolimus level is within this range, trough levels will be measured every Monday, Wednesday, and Friday or prior to the administration of the fourth dose. The target level is maintained throughout the first six (6) months posttransplantation.

Tacrolimus may be switched to cyclosporine if clinically warranted. Cyclosporine is maintained at a target level of 350–400 ng/ml. When the patient is able to take medications orally, the parenteral cyclosporine medication is changed to Neoral given every 12 h. The target level is maintained throughout the first 6 months posttransplantation. Cyclosporine trough levels are monitored in the same manner as described above for tacrolimus levels.

In the immediate postoperative period, daily monitoring of complete blood count, platelet count, liver function data, electrolytes, magnesium, calcium, phosphorus, and creatinine is performed. Frequency of blood draws is modified based on the patient's clinical condition. A baseline immune cell function level is obtained preoperatively, 1 week postoperatively, and prior to lung biopsies.

3.5 Perioperative antibiotic therapy

3.5.1 Intraoperative phase

Antibiotics are given in the operating room 1 h or less before incision and include vancomycin l g IV and cefepime 2 g IV (if allergic to penicillin, substitute ciprofloxacin 400 mg IV). Metronidazole (Flagyl) 500 mg IV is used only for patients with a history of prior *Clostridium difficile* infection.

3.5.2 Immediate postoperative phase

Postoperatively, the patient is given vancomycin 15 mg/kg IV every 12 h for 3 days (patients with a creatinine clearance of less than 50 will require renal dosing of vancomycin) and cefepime 2 g IV every 12 h for 3 days to begin 12 h after the dose given in the operating room. Ciprofloxacin 400 mg IV every 8 h for 3 days is substituted for patients with a penicillin allergy. Metronidazole (Flagyl) 500 mg IV is used only for patients with history of prior *Clostridium difficile* infection. Antibiotic therapy is adjusted by the team based on donor culture/gram stains and allergy history.

The Transplant Infectious Disease physician is consulted on all postoperative transplant patients.

3.6 Antimicrobial prophylaxis

3.6.1 Antifungal prophylaxis

Patients are ordered antifungal prophylaxis on admission to the ICU. Voriconazole (Vfend) is the first-line agent. Amphotericin B lipid complex (Abelcet) will be ordered for patients with intolerance to voriconazole (Vfend).

3.6.2 PCP prophylaxis

The patient is ordered Bactrim DS one (I) tab Monday, Wednesday, and Friday when the patient is discharged following transplant. Atovaquone (Mepron) 750 mg every 12 h is substituted or monthly inhaled pentamidine for patients with a sulfa allergy. PCP prophylaxis is given throughout the patient's posttransplant course.

3.6.3 CMV prophylaxis

Cytomegalovirus (CMV) prophylaxis is initiated on the POD# 1 based on the donor and recipient CMV status. CMV infection following the completion of the prophylaxis is treated at the induction dose for 3 weeks then decreased to the maintenance dose. Duration of therapy is determined in consultation with the Transplant Infectious Disease physician.

4. Conclusions

Lung transplantation has evolved as the gold standard for selective patients with end-stage lung disease but remains limited by a critical donor shortage. Perioperative management of lung transplant recipients is a highly complex endeavor. National registry data reveal progressively improving early as well as long-term survival. Optimal perioperative outcomes are dependent on preemptive, well-coordinated, and multidisciplinary management strategies. Certain high-risk patient subsets with end-stage lung disease such as highly sensitized patients, and those with concomitant severe CAD present unique challenges requiring specialized perioperative management.

Acknowledgements

We, the authors, would especially like to express our heartfelt gratitude to the entire lung transplant team at our institution for their professionalism, dedication, and support so generously offered to us during this endeavor.

Conflict of interest

There are no conflicts of interest.

Author details

Stacey H. Brann*, Steven S. Geier, Olga Timofeeva, Norihisa Shigemura, Francis Cordova and Yoshiya Toyoda
Temple University Hospital, Philadelphia, USA

*Address all correspondence to: stacey.brann@tuhs.temple.edu

References

[1] Yoshizumi T, Sunagawa G, Brann S, Keshavamurthy S, Dulam V, Gomez-Abraham J, et al. A study of bridge to lung transplant with extracorporeal membrane oxygenation. The Journal of Heart and Lung Transplantation. 2018;**37**(4):S253-S254

[2] Cypel M, Rubacha M, Yeung J, et al. Normothermic ex vivo perfusion prevents lung injury compared to extended cold preservation for transplantation. American Journal of Transplantation. 2009;**9**:2262-2269

[3] Ingemansson R, Eyjolfsson A, Mared L, et al. Clinical transplantation of initially rejected donor lungs after reconditioning ex vivo. The Annals of Thoracic Surgery. 2009;**87**:255-260

[4] Hayanga AJ, Aboagye JK, Hayanga H, et al. Contemporary analysis of early outcomes after lung transplantation in the elderly using a national registry. The Journal of Heart and Lung Transplantation. 2015;**34**:182-188

[5] Toyoda Y, Brann S, Keshavamurthy S, Gomez-Abraham J, Yoshizumi T, Leotta E, et al. A propensity score matched study of lung transplantation with concomitant coronary artery bypass grafting. In: Proceedings of the AATS Centennial Conference; 29 April-3 May, 2017; Boston, USA

[6] Sunagawa S, Shigemura N, Brann S, Leotta E, Kashem M, Toyoda Y. A case report of successful ECMO-bridged lung transplantation combined with off-pump coronary artery bypass grafting surgery: How should we prioritize simultaneous life-threatening urgencies? Chest. 2018;**154**(4):S1105A. DOI: 10.1016/j.chest.2018.08.1004

[7] Morrell MR, Pilewski JM, Gries CJ, et al. De novo donor-specific HLA antibodies are associated with early and high-grade bronchiolitis obliterans syndrome and death after lung transplantation. The Journal of Heart and Lung Transplantation. 2014;**33**(12):1288-1294

[8] Kulkarni HS, Bemiss BC, Hachem RR. Antibody-mediated rejection in lung transplantation. Current Transplantation Reports. 2015;**2**(4):316-323

[9] Timofeeva OA. Donor-specific HLA antibodies as biomarkers of transplant rejection. Clinics in Laboratory Medicine. 2019;**39**(1):45-60

[10] Hachem RR, Yusen RD, Meyers BF, et al. Anti-human leukocyte antigen antibodies and preemptive antibody-directed therapy after lung transplantation. The Journal of Heart and Lung Transplantation. 2010;**29**:973-980

[11] Snyder LD, Gray AL, Reynolds JM, et al. Antibody desensitization therapy in highly sensitized lung transplant candidates. The Journal of Heart and Lung Transplantation. 2014;**14**:849-856

[12] Appel JZ 3rd, Hartwig MG, Davis RD, Reinsmoen NL. Utility of peritransplant and rescue intravenous immunoglobulin and extracorporeal immunoadsorption in lung transplant recipients sensitized to HLA antigens. Human Immunology. 2005;**66**:378-386

[13] Zayek M, Hamm C, O'Donnell K, Eyal F. Induced moderate hypothermia markedly exacerbates pulmonary hypertension and dysoxia in a neonatal piglet model of elevated pulmonary vascular resistance. Critical Care. 2000;**4**(Suppl 1):P203

[14] Pasero D, Martin E, Davi A, et al. The effect of inhaled nitric oxide after lung transplantation. Minerva Anestesiologica. 2010;**76**:353-361

[15] Diamond J, Lee J, Kawut S, et al. Clinical risk factors for primary graft dysfunction after lung transplantation. American Journal of Respiratory and Critical Care Medicine. 2013;**187**:527-534

[16] Eberlein M, Reed R, Bolukbas S, et al. Lung size mismatch and primary graft dysfunction after bilateral lung transplantation. The Journal of Heart and Lung Transplantation. 2015;**34**:233-240

[17] Dezube R, Arnaoutakis G, Reed R, et al. The effect of lung-size mismatch on mechanical ventilation tidal volumes after bilateral lung transplantation. Interactive CardioVascular and Thoracic Surgery. 2013;**16**:275-281

[18] Christie J, Carby M, Bag R, et al. Report of the ISHLT working group on primary graft dysfunction part II: Definition. A consensus statement of the International Society for Heart and Lung Transplantation. The Journal of Heart and Lung Transplantation. 2005;**24**(10):1454-1459

[19] Gelman A, Fisher A, Huang H, et al. Report of the ISHLT working group on primary graft dysfunction part III: Mechanisms. A 2016 consensus group statement of the International Society of Heart and Lung Transplantation. The Journal of Heart and Lung Transplantation. 2017;**36**(10):1115-1120

[20] Prekker M, Herrington C, Hertz M, et al. Early trends in PaO_2/fraction of inspired oxygen ratio predict outcome in lung transplant recipients with severe primary graft dysfunction. Chest. 2007;**132**(3):991-997

[21] Arcasoy S, Fisher A, Hachem R, et al. Report of the ISHLT working group on primary graft dysfunction part V: Predictors and outcomes. The Journal of Heart and Lung Transplantation. 2005;**24**(10):1451-1453; 2017;**36**(10):1115-1120

[22] Raemdonck D, Matthew H, Hertz M, et al. Report of the ISHLT working group on primary graft dysfunction part IV: Prevention and treatment: A 2016 consensus group statement of the International Society for Heart and Lung Transplantation. The Journal of Heart and Lung Transplantation. 2017;**36**(10):1121-1136

[23] Currey J, Pilcher D, Davies A, et al. Implementation of a management guidelines aimed at minimizing the severity of primary graft dysfunction after lung transplant. The Journal of Thoracic and Cardiovascular Surgery. 2010;**139**:154-161

[24] Nagendran M, Maruthappu M, Sugand K. Should double lung transplant be performed with or without cardiopulmonary bypass? Interactive Cardiovasc Thorac Surg. 2012;**12**:799-805

[25] Wang Y, Kurichi J, Blumenthal N, et al. Multiple variables affecting blood usage in lung transplantation. The Journal of Heart and Lung Transplantation. 2006;**25**:533-538; 2017;**36**(10):1115-1120

[26] Visentin J, Marroc M, Guidicelli G, et al. Clinical impact of preformed donor-specific denatured class I HLA antibodies after kidney transplantation. Clinical Transplantation. 2015;**29**(5):393-402

[27] Visentin J, Guidicelli G, Moreau JF, Lee JH, Taupin JL. Deciphering allogeneic antibody response against native and denatured HLA epitopes in organ transplantation. European Journal of Immunology. 2015;**45**(7):2111-2121

[28] Oaks M, Michel K, Sulemanjee NZ, Thohan V, Downey FX. Practical value of identifying antibodies to cryptic HLA epitopes in cardiac transplantation. The Journal of Heart and Lung Transplantation. 2014;**33**(7):713-720

[29] Grenzi PC, de Marco R, Silva RZ, Campos EF, Gerbase-DeLima M. Antibodies against denatured HLA class II molecules detected in luminex-single antigen assay. Human Immunology. 2013;**74**(10):1300-1303

[30] Jucaud V, Ravindranath MH, Terasaki PI. Conformational variants of the individual HLA-I antigens on Luminex single antigen beads used in monitoring HLA antibodies: Problems and solutions. Transplantation. 2017;**101**(4):764-777

[31] Timofeeva O, Kashem M, Geier S, Grogan D, Keshavamurthy S, Gomez-Abraham J, et al. Eliminating false positive virtual Crossmatch results for lung transplant candidates by using multiple antibody testing platforms. American Journal of Transplantation. Apr 2017;**17**(suppl 3):595. DOI: 10.1111/ajt.14304

[32] Courtwright A, Diamond JM, Wood I, et al. Detection and clinical impact of human leukocyte antigen antibodies in lung transplantation: A systematic review and meta-analysis. HLA. 2018;**91**(2):102-111

[33] Tambur AR, Campbell P, Claas FH, et al. Sensitization in transplantation: Assessment of risk (STAR) 2017 working group meeting report. American Journal of Transplantation. 2018;**18**(7):1604-1614

[34] Tinckam KJ, Keshavjee S, Chaparro C, et al. Survival in sensitized lung transplant recipients with perioperative desensitization. American Journal of Transplantation. 2015;**15**(2):417-426

Chapter 6

Cytokine Biomarkers as Indicators of Primary Graft Dysfunction, Acute Rejection, and Chronic Lung Allograft Dysfunction in Lung Transplant Recipients: A Review

John Hallsten and Wickii T. Vigneswaran

Abstract

Lung transplantation is well accepted form of treatment for end-stage lung disease in selected patients. The number of lung transplants performed worldwide has increased annually with chronic obstructive pulmonary disease being the leading cause. The morbidity and mortality in the early period are due to nonspecific primary graft dysfunction (PGD) and acute lung rejection (ALR). Chronic lung allograft dysfunction (CLAD) is the cause of long-term complications following lung transplantation and seen in almost half of the patient during the first 5 years. Activation of pro- and anti-inflammatory cytokines and chemokines has been described during various phases of lung transplantation recovery. We reviewed the literature for cytokine activity associated with PGD, ALR, and CLAD. This review aims to summarize the specific associations between bronchoalveolar lavage (BAL) and plasma cytokine levels and the association of PGD, ALR, and CLAD.

Keywords: cytokines, lung transplant, primary graft dysfunction, acute rejection, chronic lung allograft dysfunction

1. Introduction

The incidence of lung transplantations worldwide has increased annually with chronic obstructive pulmonary disease being the leading cause [1]. From 2009 to June 2016, the median survival of primary lung transplantation was 6.5 years [2]. The frequency of at least one treated acute rejection episode occurring within 1 year posttransplantation is around 27% [2]. Bronchiolitis obliterans syndrome (BOS), a phenotype of chronic lung rejection, is currently one of the most significant long-term complications of lung transplantation with a 5-year follow-up incidence of 41.5% [2].

Primary graft dysfunction (PGD) complicates lung transplant outcomes. PGD is a common early complication of lung transplantation that often occurs in the first

72 h posttransplantation [3]. PGD has also been indicated as a risk factor for the development of BOS [4].

Acute lung rejection (ALR) in lung transplant recipients is a major cause of early complication and death [5]. It is a major risk factor for the development of BOS [6]. BOS is the most common manifestation of chronic lung allograft dysfunction (CLAD) and is characterized by subepithelial fibrosis of small cartilaginous airways leading to partial or total occlusion [7].

PGD, ALR, and CLAD all have been associated with pro- and anti-inflammatory cytokine and chemokine expressions. This review aims to summarize the specific associations between bronchoalveolar lavage (BAL) and plasma cytokine levels and the development of PGD, ALR, and CLAD.

2. Methods

PubMed was explored using MeSH terms "lung transplantation," "cytokines," "biomarkers," "acute rejection," "chronic allograft dysfunction," and "primary graft dysfunction." Inclusion criteria consisted of studies through May 2018 that provided information on plasma and/or BAL cytokines and acute rejection, chronic rejection, or primary graft dysfunction in lung transplant recipients. Prospective, retrospective, and review articles were included. The references of searched articles were also examined for potential studies to include. We focused on the following cytokines: interleukin (IL)-1a, IL-1b, IL-2, IL-4, IL-6, IL-8, IL-10, IL-12, IL-15, and IL-17; interferon-gamma (IFN-y); tumor necrosis factor-alpha (TNF-a); transforming growth factor-beta (TGF-b); and monocyte chemotactic protein (MCP)-1.

3. Primary graft dysfunction

PGD typically occurs within the first 72 h posttransplantation and is identified as ischemia-reperfusion injury with pulmonary edema that presents as increasing hypoxia in the affected patient [3].

Lung transplantation, and any other major surgeries, constitutes massive damage to patient tissues.

TNF-α is one of the first cytokines to be released into circulation from such an injury, peaking in serum concentration around 1 h after the beginning of injury. IL-6, IL-8, and IL-10 are expressed and released in circulation shortly after, with peaks in concentration between 2 and 4 h after injury. Additionally, if injury severity increases, there is an associated shift away from a cell-mediated response to a humoral immune response [8].

Macrophage-associated cytokines IFN-y, TNF-a, and MCP-1 have all been strongly associated with PGD development in lung transplant recipients. Bharat and associates identified elevated serum IFN-γ in PGD positive patients [9]. Early release of TNF-α was associated with early hemodynamic failure posttransplantation [10]. In another study, elevated systemic TNF-α concentrations were associated with PGD development [11]. MCP-1, a macrophage chemotactic agent, has demonstrated a strong role in PGD. Shah and associates measured plasma MCP-1 at various time points in lung transplant recipients. They found elevated MCP-1 levels at 24 h posttransplantation were associated with PGD grade 3. These results attested to the importance of monocyte chemotaxis in PGD [12]. Another group of authors found similar results with elevated serum MCP-1 in PGD positive lung transplant recipients [13]. INF-γ is a potent activator of macrophages. Elevations in IFN-γ along with increases in MCP-1, a strong monocyte chemotactic agent, suggest that ischemia-reperfusion injury increases macrophage activation.

Macrophage activation leads to release of pro-inflammatory cytokines, including IL-6 and IL-8. PGD is linked to concomitant increases in IL-6 and IL-8 in lung transplant recipients. Early hemodynamic failure posttransplantation was associated with increases in both IL-6 and IL-8 [10]. A different study had similar results, in which IL-6 and IL-8 were both elevated in patients with PGD [11]. Moreno and associates found elevated BAL and blood IL-6 and IL-8 in patients with PGD. They are subsequently treated with inhaled nitric oxide, which lowered IL-6 and IL-8 and also decreased PGD incidence [14]. Increases in IL-6 often occur as a result of upstream macrophage-induced activation of Th1 immunity. In addition to macrophage activation, neutrophil chemotaxis from IL-8 upregulation is associated with increased PGD incidence. Increases in other pro-inflammatory cytokines caused by macrophage activation lead to pulmonary vasoconstriction and increased pulmonary vascular permeability, precipitating hemodynamic instability characteristic of PGD.

4. Acute lung rejection

In the weeks to months following transplantation, the allograft recipient's T-cell-mediated immunity intensifies, potentially leading to the development of ALR. ALR is understood to be originally caused by mismatched MHC recognition and adaptive immune response [15].

Acute lung rejection is precipitated by the adaptive T-cell response. MHC mismatch and the adaptive immune response are associated with T-cell activation and differentiation, which is facilitated by IL-2 [16]. It is expected that IL-2 would be increased in acute rejection; however the literature is conflicting on its association with lung rejection. Jordan and associates analyzed the serum of 17 lung transplant recipients and found serum IL-2 significantly elevated in patients with acute rejection confirmed; however, Moudgil and associates found no correlation between IL-2 levels and acute rejection in lung transplant recipient [17, 18]. In addition to IL-2, IL-15 is a cytokine derived from stromal cells that behaves similarly to IL-2 in terms of biological function and is involved in T-cell chemoattraction to allografts [23]. Bhorade and associates measured IL-15 levels in BAL fluid of lung transplants and found that IL-15 was significantly elevated in patients experiencing acute rejection when the patients were given anti-CD25 monoclonal antibodies [19]. This study along with the evidence for IL-2 activation suggests the potential importance of IL-2 and IL-2 receptors in ALR immune responses.

T helper (Th) cells orchestrate the immune response and are divided into two subsets, Th1 and Th2 cells. T-cell differentiation into Th1 cells leads to increased expression of IFN-γ by Th1 cells. IFN-γ is involved in many important immune mechanisms and is a main component of the Th1 immune response, as it is a strong activator of macrophage-mediated antimicrobial and antitumor activity [20]. Its role in ALR is supported by a study measuring IFN-γ in BAL fluid of lung transplantation patients, which found IFN-γ levels were significantly elevated in early acute rejection [18]. IL-12 is a known mediator of interferon-gamma expression [21]. D'ovidio and associates found IL-12 in BAL fluid elevated in acute rejection patients, which suggests it influences IFN-γ in ALR [22]. Ultimately, IFN-γ activation of macrophages induces pro-inflammatory cytokine release to cause inflammation.

IL-1, IL-6, and TNF-α are all acute phase pro-inflammatory cytokines that occur in most disease states and are secreted by activated macrophages to induce inflammation. IL-1, which consists of both IL-1a and IL-1b, is a ubiquitous cytoplasmic cytokine that is associated with a plethora of disease states, including allograft rejection [23]. This family is associated with general acute phase reactions. Because the IL-1 family has been linked to several disease states, it is no surprise that lung transplant rejection bears an association to its expression. Specifically, Patella and associates recently found BAL IL-1β elevated in acute rejection episodes [24]. In another study, Rizzo and associates found significant increases in IL-1a and IL-1b expressions from alveolar macrophages of acute lung rejection patients compared to patients without acute rejection [25]. IL-6 is another acute phase marker and pro-inflammatory cytokine that is involved in hematopoiesis and immune regulation [26]. Its role in immunity is similar to that of IL-1 cytokines, which leads it to also be elevated in acute rejection. The literature supports this claim. Whitehead and associates also found IL-6 significantly elevated in the BAL of acute lung rejection patients [27]. Patella and associates examined IL-6 in BAL samples of lung transplant recipients and found IL-6 to be higher in acute rejection cases [24]. The last of the acute phase cytokines is TNF-a. TNF-α has been associated with many disease processes, including infections, septic shock, and allograft rejection [28]. Hodge and associates found TNF-α was elevated in BAL CD4+ and CD8+ cells in acute lung rejection cases [29]. Magnan and associates measured TNF-α in alveolar macrophages and lung transplant recipients and found increased TNF-α in acute rejection [30].

In addition to acute phase cytokines, IL-8 is a known mediator of inflammation and neutrophil chemotaxis [31]. Its role in ALR, however, is minor. A recent study found no association between IL-8 and acute rejection [22].

Along with Th1, Th2 differentiation occurs with IL-2 activation of naive T cells. In addition, Th2 cell differentiation is activated by IL-4, a cytokine normally released by mast cells and basophils [32]. The literature is currently conflicting on the role of IL-4 in acute lung rejection. Whitehead and associates found BAL IL-4 elevated in acute lung rejection patients compared to patients without rejection [27]. On the other hand, another study looking at pro-inflammatory cytokine expression in lung transplant recipients found no difference in BAL, plasma, or bronchial brushing IL-4 levels between acute rejection and stable patients [29]. Based on conflicting literature, the Th2 response may not have a significant role in acute lung rejection.

The Th1 response is regulated by anti-inflammatory cytokines. IL-10 is an anti-inflammatory cytokine that is involved in immune response regulation and limiting of immune destruction to host tissues [33]. Patella and associates found that IL-10 was actually elevated in acute rejection cases compared to stable patients [24]. This evidence suggests IL-10 is elevated in an attempt to limit inflammation in ALR.

Monocyte and macrophage activity is strongly associated with activation of the Th1 response and is responsible for secretion of pro-inflammatory cytokines. IL-17, also known as IL-17A, is released by Th17 cells and induces monocytes and stromal cells to produce cytokines in addition to stimulating granulopoiesis. It is also involved in the pathogenesis of several autoimmune diseases [34]. In a study analyzed IL-17 mRNA and protein levels in BAL samples of lung transplant recipients, the authors found both IL-17 mRNA and protein levels significantly elevated in acute lung rejection [35]. MCP-1, also known as CCL-2, is a chemokine with strong mononuclear cell chemotaxis properties involved in chronic inflammation [36]. Belperio and associates evaluated BAL fluid from lung transplant recipients and found increased levels of MCP-1 in acute rejection cases compared to stable patients [37]. The role of MCP-1 and IL-17 suggest that mononuclear immune cell regulation occurs concomitantly to the Th1 response in ALR.

5. Chronic lung allograft dysfunction

Airway inflammation is the main contributor to CLAD. CLAD encompasses many manifestations of chronic rejection, including BOS and RAS (restrictive allograft syndrome). Currently, it is characterized by a decrease in FEV_1 and/or FVC by at least 20% compared to baseline, which is determined as a mean of two optimal postoperative measurements taken 3 weeks apart [38].

Pro-inflammatory cytokines IL-1, IL-6, and TNF-α are all upregulated in CLAD. Firstly, IL-1 has been studied in the setting of chronic rejection in lung transplantation. Suwara and associates studied cytokine expression in BAL fluid of lung transplant recipients with respect to different phenotypes of CLAD. They found IL-1a and IL-1b were elevated in lymphocytic bronchiolitis and persistent airway neutrophilia cases [39]. Verleden and associates also analyzed BAL fluid cytokines in different chronic lung rejection phenotypes and found IL-1b was significantly elevated in neutrophilic BOS and RAS episodes compared to stable patients [40]. In persistent airway neutrophilia, a specific phenotype of CLAD, BAL IL-6 was found to be significantly elevated [39]. Verleden and associates studied cytokine expression in BAL fluid of lung transplant recipients and found that IL-6 levels were elevated in RAS patient and correlated with survival among lung transplantation patients with RAS [40]. Lastly, TNF-α has been linked to CLAD. Suwara and associates studied cytokine expression in the context of several CLAD phenotypes. They found that BAL TNF-α levels were increased in patients with primary airway neutrophilia [39]. Additionally, Bharat and associates measured serum cytokines in patients with and without BOS after lung transplantations. They found that IL-10 *decreased* threefold during the onset of BOS [41]. This evidence suggests that inflammation in the absence of regulation may contribute to airway inflammation in CLAD which likely arises from uninhibited pro-inflammatory cytokines.

Pro-inflammatory cytokine expression in CLAD may be a result of increased monocyte/macrophage chemotaxis. IFN-y, which activates macrophages to induce inflammation, has been indicated in chronic lung rejection. Hodge and associates found that, compared to BOS patients, stable lung transplant recipients displayed significant reductions in blood IFN-γ levels [42]. Both IL-17 and MCP-1, which are macrophage-recruiting cytokines, have been indicated in CLAD. MCP-1 was found elevated in patients before and during BOS indicating elevated MCP-1 posttransplantation is predictive of BOS [13]. Fisichella and associates found increases in BAL IL-17 as an indicator of early onset BOS [43].

Unlike ALR, neutrophil-associated airway damage is strongly associated with CLAD development. IL-8 is known to facilitate neutrophil chemotaxis and has shown to be involved in chronic rejection among lung transplant recipients. DiGiovine and associates first established the contribution of IL-8 expression to airway neutrophilia and BOS development [44]. BAL IL-8 levels in lung transplantation patients were elevated in neutrophilic BOS and RAS compared to stable patients in a recent study [40]. Elssner and associates found that IL-8 mRNA expression from bronchial cells was significantly elevated in BOS cases compared to stable patients [45].

The activity of IL-12 in CLAD is also contrary to ALR. IL-12 appears to attenuate the development of CLAD, specifically BOS. Meloni and associates measured BAL cytokines in 44 lung transplant recipients and identified significant decreases in IL-12 to be correlative with BOS development [46]. Krenn and associates determined that azithromycin administration in lung transplant recipients reduced overall fibrosis and kept IL-12 levels from decreasing [47]. The authors remarked on the future significance of macrolide therapy in reduction of BOS development through effects on IL-12. The Th2 cytokine IL-4 has also shown to contribute to CLAD. Kastelijn and associates measured serum IL-4 levels in lung transplant recipients and found IL-4 levels were significantly lower in patients with BOS than BOS-negative patients [48]. The importance of IL-12 as a negative regulator as well as the potential role of IL-4 in CLAD indicates that the Th1 response may be downregulated in CLAD.

Chronic inflammation from persistent airway damage eventually leads to airway remodeling. TGF-β is an anti-inflammatory cytokine involved in tissue remodeling and scar formation [49]. Several studies have correlated TGF-β with the development of chronic lung rejection episodes, including El-Gamel and associates who discovered elevated TGF-β levels in biopsies in patients with BOS [50]. Elssner and associates studied BAL fluid and respiratory epithelial lining fluid in lung transplant recipients and found that BOS patients had elevated TGF-β levels in both samples [45]. Another study correlated TGF-β levels with BOS, which validated the author's claims that the biological role of TGF-β in tissue repair may also lead to airway fibrosis and obliteration [51].

6. Conclusions

The literature contains ample evidence on cytokines as biomarkers in lung transplantation outcomes. PGD is augmented by IFN-y, IL-6, IL-8, TNF-a, and MCP-1. This could be explained by monocyte involvement and inflammatory changes during ischemia-reperfusion injury. IL-1b, IL-6, IL-10, IL-15, and IFN-γ appear to be strong indicators to supplement the diagnosis of acute rejection in lung transplant recipients. These cytokines are linked to a Th1 immune response associated with acute inflammation. IL-1b, IL-6, IL8, IL-15, IL-17, IFN-γ, and TGF-β are significant contributors to chronic lung allograft dysfunction. IL-12 has also shown to attenuate chronic lung rejection. CLAD appears to be more associated with inflammation and airway neutrophil chemotaxis.

The role of cytokines requires more controlled studies in order for diagnostic characteristics to be attributed. That being said, cytokines and chemokines in primary graft dysfunction, acute rejection, and chronic allograft dysfunction are promising markers of future diagnostic tests and targets of therapies to ultimately improve outcomes and survival in lung transplant recipients.

Author details

John Hallsten and Wickii T. Vigneswaran*
Department of Thoracic and Cardiovascular Surgery, Loyola University Health System, Maywood, IL, USA

*Address all correspondence to: wickii.vigneswaran@lumc.edu

References

[1] Yusen RD, Edwards LB, Dipchand AI, et al. The registry of the international society for heart and lung transplantation: Thirty-third adult lung and heart-lung transplant report-2016; focus theme: Primary diagnostic indications for transplant. The Journal of Heart and Lung Transplantation. 2016;**35**:1170-1184

[2] Chambers DC, Cherikh WS, Goldfarb SB, et al. The international thoracic organ transplant registry of the international society for heart and lung transplantation: Thirty-fifth adult lung and heart-lung transplant report-2018; focus theme: Multiorgan transplantation. The Journal of Heart and Lung Transplantation. 2018;**37**:1169-1183

[3] de Perrot M, Liu M, Waddell TK, Keshavjee S. Ischemia-reperfusion-induced lung injury. American Journal of Respiratory and Critical Care Medicine. 2003;**167**:490-511

[4] Huang HJ, Yusen RD, Meyers BF, et al. Late primary graft dysfunction after lung transplantation and bronchiolitis obliterans syndrome. American Journal of Transplantation. 2008;**8**:2454-2462

[5] Sundaresan S, Alevy YG, Steward N, et al. Cytokine gene transcripts for tumor necrosis factor-alpha, interleukin-2, and interferon-gamma in human pulmonary allografts. The Journal of Heart and Lung Transplantation. 1995;**14**:512-518

[6] Greenland JR, Jones KD, Hays SR, et al. Association of large-airway lymphocytic bronchitis with bronchiolitis obliterans syndrome. American Journal of Respiratory and Critical Care Medicine. 2013;**187**:417-423

[7] Stewart S, Fishbein MC, Snell GI, et al. Revision of the 1996 working formulation for the standardization of nomenclature in the diagnosis of lung rejection. The Journal of Heart and Lung Transplantation. 2007;**26**:1229-1242

[8] Baigrie RJ, Lamont PM, Kwiatkowski D, Dallman MJ, Morris PJ. Systemic cytokine response after major surgery. The British Journal of Surgery. 1992;**79**:757-760

[9] Bharat A, Kuo E, Steward N, et al. Immunological link between primary graft dysfunction and chronic lung allograft rejection. The Annals of Thoracic Surgery. 2008;**86**:7

[10] Mal H, Dehoux M, Sleiman C, et al. Early release of proinflammatory cytokines after lung transplantation. Chest. 1998;**113**:645-651

[11] Mathur A, Baz M, Staples ED, et al. Cytokine profile after lung transplantation: Correlation with allograft injury. The Annals of Thoracic Surgery. 2006;**81**:50

[12] Shah RJ, Diamond JM, Lederer DJ, et al. Plasma monocyte chemotactic protein-1 levels at 24 hours are a biomarker of primary graft dysfunction after lung transplantation. Translational Research. 2012;**160**:435-442

[13] Reynaud-Gaubert M, Marin V, Thirion X, et al. Upregulation of chemokines in bronchoalveolar lavage fluid as a predictive marker of post-transplant airway obliteration. The Journal of Heart and Lung Transplantation. 2002;**21**:721-730

[14] Moreno I, Mir A, Vicente R, et al. Analysis of interleukin-6 and interleukin-8 in lung transplantation: Correlation with nitric oxide administration. Transplantation Proceedings. 2008;**40**:3082-3084

[15] Taylor AL, Watson CJ, Bradley JA. Immunosuppressive agents in solid organ transplantation: Mechanisms of action and therapeutic efficacy. Critical Reviews in Oncology/Hematology. 2005;**56**:23-46

[16] Paul WE, Seder RA. Lymphocyte responses and cytokines. Cell. 1994;**76**:241-251

[17] Jordan SC, Marchevski A, Ross D, Toyoda M, Waters PF. Serum interleukin-2 levels in lung transplant recipients: Correlation with findings on transbronchial biopsy. The Journal of Heart and Lung Transplantation. 1992;**11**:1001-1004

[18] Moudgil A, Bagga A, Toyoda M, Nicolaidou E, Jordan SC, Ross D. Expression of gamma-IFN mRNA in bronchoalveolar lavage fluid correlates with early acute allograft rejection in lung transplant recipients. Clinical Transplantation. 1999;**13**:201-207

[19] Bhorade SM, Yu A, Vigneswaran WT, Alex CG, Garrity ER. Elevation of interleukin-15 protein expression in bronchoalveolar fluid in acute lung allograft rejection. Chest. 2007;**131**:533-538

[20] Schroder K, Hertzog PJ, Ravasi T, Hume DA. Interferon-gamma: An overview of signals, mechanisms and functions. Journal of Leukocyte Biology. 2004;**75**:163-189

[21] Keane MP, Belperio JA, Burdick MD, Strieter RM. IL-12 attenuates bleomycin-induced pulmonary fibrosis. American Journal of Physiology. Lung Cellular and Molecular Physiology. 2001;**281**:92

[22] D'Ovidio F, Kaneda H, Chaparro C, et al. Pilot study exploring lung allograft surfactant protein A (SP-A) expression in association with lung transplant outcome. American Journal of Transplantation. 2013;**13**:2722-2729

[23] Dinarello CA. Biologic basis for interleukin-1 in disease. Blood. 1996;**87**:2095-2147

[24] Patella M, Anile M, Del Porto P, et al. Role of cytokine profile in the differential diagnosis between acute lung rejection and pulmonary infections after lung transplantationdagger. European Journal of Cardio-Thoracic Surgery. 2015;**47**:1031-1036

[25] Rizzo M, SivaSai KS, Smith MA, et al. Increased expression of inflammatory cytokines and adhesion molecules by alveolar macrophages of human lung allograft recipients with acute rejection: Decline with resolution of rejection. The Journal of Heart and Lung Transplantation. 2000;**19**:858-865

[26] Tanaka T, Narazaki M, Kishimoto T. IL-6 in inflammation, immunity, and disease. Cold Spring Harbor Perspectives in Biology. 2014;**6**:a016295

[27] Whitehead BF, Stoehr C, Wu CJ, et al. Cytokine gene expression in human lung transplant recipients. Transplantation. 1993;**56**:956-961

[28] Strieter RM, Kunkel SL, Bone RC. Role of tumor necrosis factor-alpha in disease states and inflammation. Critical Care Medicine. 1993;**21**:447

[29] Hodge G, Hodge S, Chambers D, Reynolds PN, Holmes M. Acute lung transplant rejection is associated with localized increase in T-cell IFNgamma and TNFalpha proinflammatory cytokines in the airways. Transplantation. 2007;**84**:1452-1458

[30] Magnan A, Mege JL, Reynaud M, et al. Monitoring of alveolar macrophage production of tumor necrosis factor-alpha and interleukin-6 in lung transplant recipients. Marseille and Montreal Lung Transplantation Group. American Journal of Respiratory and Critical Care Medicine. 1994;**150**:684-689

[31] Allen TC, Kurdowska A. Interleukin 8 and acute lung injury. Archives of Pathology & Laboratory Medicine. 2014;**138**:266-269

[32] Mowen KA, Glimcher LH. Signaling pathways in Th2 development. Immunological Reviews. 2004;**202**:203-222

[33] Moore KW, de Waal Malefyt R, Coffman RL, O'Garra A. Interleukin-10 and the interleukin-10 receptor. Annual Review of Immunology. 2001;**19**:683-765

[34] Shilling RA, Wilkes DS. Role of Th17 cells and IL-17 in lung transplant rejection. Seminars in Immunopathology. 2011;**33**:129-134

[35] Vanaudenaerde BM, Dupont LJ, Wuyts WA, et al. The role of interleukin-17 during acute rejection after lung transplantation. The European Respiratory Journal. 2006;**27**:779-787

[36] Gong JH, Ratkay LG, Waterfield JD, Clark-Lewis I. An antagonist of monocyte chemoattractant protein 1 (MCP-1) inhibits arthritis in the MRL-lpr mouse model. The Journal of Experimental Medicine. 1997;**186**:131-137

[37] Belperio JA, Keane MP, Burdick MD, et al. Critical role for the chemokine MCP-1/CCR2 in the pathogenesis of bronchiolitis obliterans syndrome. The Journal of Clinical Investigation. 2001;**108**:547-556

[38] Verleden GM, Raghu G, Meyer KC, Glanville AR, Corris P. A new classification system for chronic lung allograft dysfunction. The Journal of Heart and Lung Transplantation. 2014;**33**:127-133

[39] Suwara MI, Vanaudenaerde BM, Verleden SE, et al. Mechanistic differences between phenotypes of chronic lung allograft dysfunction after lung transplantation. Transplant International. 2014;**27**:857-867

[40] Verleden SE, Ruttens D, Vos R, et al. Differential cytokine, chemokine and growth factor expression in phenotypes of chronic lung allograft dysfunction. Transplantation. 2015;**99**:86-93

[41] Bharat A, Narayanan K, Street T, et al. Early posttransplant inflammation promotes the development of alloimmunity and chronic human lung allograft rejection. Transplantation. 2007;**83**:150-158

[42] Hodge G, Hodge S, Chambers D, Reynolds PN, Holmes M. Bronchiolitis obliterans syndrome is associated with absence of suppression of peripheral blood Th1 proinflammatory cytokines. Transplantation. 2009;**88**:211-218

[43] Fisichella PM, Davis CS, Lowery E, Ramirez L, Gamelli RL, Kovacs EJ. Aspiration, localized pulmonary inflammation, and predictors of early-onset bronchiolitis obliterans syndrome after lung transplantation. Journal of the American College of Surgeons. 2013;**217**:1

[44] DiGiovine B, Lynch JP 3rd, Martinez FJ, et al. Bronchoalveolar lavage neutrophilia is associated with obliterative bronchiolitis after lung transplantation: Role of IL-8. Journal of Immunology. 1996;**157**:4194-4202

[45] Elssner A, Jaumann F, Dobmann S, et al. Elevated levels of interleukin-8 and transforming growth factor-beta in bronchoalveolar lavage fluid from patients with bronchiolitis obliterans syndrome: Proinflammatory role of bronchial epithelial cells. Munich Lung Transplant Group. Transplantation. 2000;**70**:362-367

[46] Meloni F, Vitulo P, Cascina A, et al. Bronchoalveolar lavage cytokine profile in a cohort of lung transplant recipients:

A predictive role of interleukin-12 with respect to onset of bronchiolitis obliterans syndrome. The Journal of Heart and Lung Transplantation. 2004;**23**:1053-1060

[47] Krenn K, Gmeiner M, Paulus P, et al. Effects of azithromycin and tanomastat on experimental bronchiolitis obliterans. The Journal of Thoracic and Cardiovascular Surgery. 2015;**149**:1194-1202

[48] Kastelijn EA, Rijkers GT, Van Moorsel CH, et al. Systemic and exhaled cytokine and chemokine profiles are associated with the development of bronchiolitis obliterans syndrome. The Journal of Heart and Lung Transplantation. 2010;**29**:997-1008

[49] Clark DA, Coker R. Transforming growth factor-beta (TGF-beta). The International Journal of Biochemistry & Cell Biology. 1998;**30**:293-298

[50] El-Gamel A, Sim E, Hasleton P, et al. Transforming growth factor beta (TGF-beta) and obliterative bronchiolitis following pulmonary transplantation. The Journal of Heart and Lung Transplantation. 1999;**18**:828-837

[51] DerHovanessian A, Weigt SS, Palchevskiy V, et al. The role of TGF-beta in the association between primary graft dysfunction and bronchiolitis obliterans syndrome. American Journal of Transplantation. 2016;**16**:640-649

Section 4

Transplant Recipient - Postoperative Mental Dysfunction

Chapter 7

Delirium Management, Treatment and Prevention Solid Organ Transplantation

Clark D. Kensinger and Jon S. Odorico

Abstract

Delirium following solid organ transplant is a very common complication. Post-operative delirium has been shown to be associated with longer length of stays, increased post-operative complications, increased readmission rates, higher costs, and increased mortality. Therefore, every healthcare provider who is involved in the care of transplant recipients should be well educated in the importance of early diagnosis of delirium, treatment of potential contributing factors, and optimizing management. Routine delirium screening to allow prompt diagnosis and workup is paramount to the care of post-operative transplant patients. Identifying high risk individuals for pre-operative rehabilitation to help decrease post-operative delirium rates, as well as focusing on functional and cognitive recovery following delirium are important preventative and rehabilitation efforts to optimize outcomes for transplant patients. This chapter will highlight a proactive approach to delirium prevention and management in the transplant population.

Keywords: delirium, outcomes, complications, altered mental status, solid organ transplant, cognitive impairment

1. Introduction

Delirium following transplantation is a wide reaching problem that has a significant effect on recovery time, functional outcomes, and has a profound economic impact on the healthcare system. Delirium is now being recognized as a major driver of poor health care related outcomes. Post-operative delirium has been shown to be associated with longer length of stays, increased post-operative complications, increased readmission rates, higher costs, longer periods of mechanical ventilation, prolonged cognitive impairment and increased mortality [1, 2]. With this in mind, early diagnosis of delirium, treatment of potential contributing factors, and optimized management is paramount to improve post-transplant outcomes. This chapter will highlight a proactive approach to delirium management and prevention in the abdominal transplant population.

1.1 Definition

Delirium is defined as a condition highlighted by an acute disturbance in attention, awareness and cognition that is not explained by a preexisting neurocognitive disorder. Delirium is characterized by reduced capacity to direct, focus, sustain, or shift attention, as well as reduced orientation to the environment [1, 3]. These symptoms must present acutely and fluctuate throughout the day. Importantly, the diagnosis of delirium identifies the constellation of symptoms representing altered brain function, but does not identify the etiology (**Figure 1**).

Delirium can be classified into three subtypes based on psychomotor behavior: hyperactive, hypoactive and mixed type delirium. Delirium is under diagnosed due to inconsistent screening, but also because delirium has varying and inconsistent presentations especially in patients suffering from hypoactive delirium. Hypoactive delirium is characterized by slowed mentation, lethargy, and decreased movement, whereas hyperactive delirium is marked by agitated behavior, confusion and difficulty with re-orientation. Without consistent, evidence-based screening methods, hypoactive delirium is more likely to be overlooked compared to hyperactive delirium. In addition, the different forms of delirium carry different prognosis. In a study of patients admitted to the intensive care unit after elective operations, patients that suffered from hypoactive delirium had an increased six-month mortality compared to patients with other subtypes of delirium (32 vs. 8.7%, $P = 0.04$) [4]. Therefore, it is important understand the various forms of delirium and the clinical scenarios in which it can present to allow timely diagnosis and management.

1.2 Prevalence

The prevalence of delirium is highly variable based on the population being evaluated. It has been reported to occur in 16–89% of hospitalized patients, and up to 50% of post-operative patients [5, 6]. Delirium is the most common manifestation of acute brain dysfunction during critical illness. Reports note that delirium affects 50–75% of patients who receive medical ventilation in the intensive care unit [5]. The prevalence in the transplant population has been reported to range from 12 to 47% of patients [7]. Patients undergoing liver transplant have a higher prevalence of developing delirium than other abdominal transplant recipients occurring in

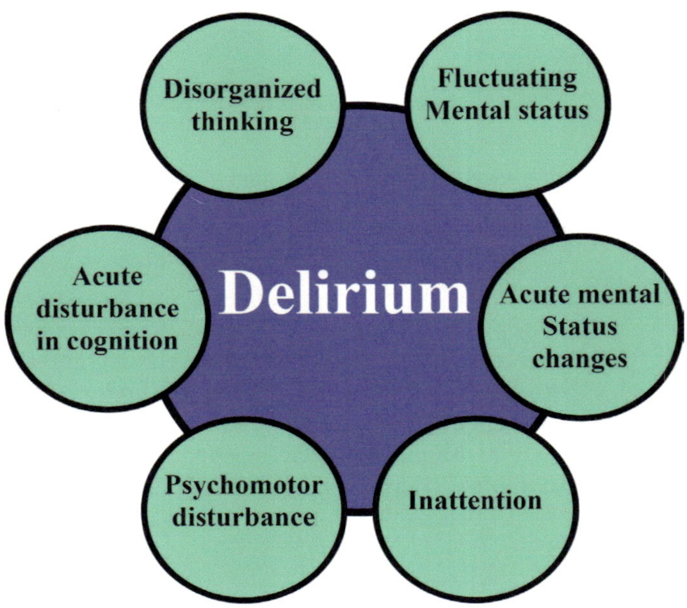

Figure 1.
Clinical symptomatology associated with delirium.

approximately 45% of the liver recipients [8]. In a recent report by Haugen et al. only 0.8% of kidneys transplant recipients developed delirium [9]. The difference in prevalence of delirium in abdominal transplant recipients needs to be considered when developing preventive strategies to provide targeted interventions on high-risk populations.

1.3 Pathophysiology

The pathophysiology associated with delirium development is multifactorial and is associated with complex interactions between systemic and cerebral physiology. The precise mechanisms are still being investigated, however many hypotheses exist for the underlying precipitating factor(s) that lead to delirium development. Examples of different hypotheses include inflammatory-mediated neuronal injury, altered cerebral perfusion, increased permeability of the blood brain barrier from endothelial dysfunction, and altered neurotransmitter balance [10]. In addition, the anatomic changes associated with advanced age including cerebral atrophy and changes in white matter density have been considered to contribute to the underlying mechanism of delirium, and also represent risk factors for delirium development [11].

Delirium pathophysiology is also believed to be associated with the systemic inflammatory cascade that occurs as a result of the stress response following an acute event, trauma or surgical intervention. The release of inflammatory mediators and cytokines (cortisol, c-reactive protein, interleukin-6, interleukin-8, etc.) following surgery likely play a significant role in the pathophysiologic link between surgery and delirium development [10]. Microglial cells have an intimate involvement in mediating the cerebral inflammatory response that occurs as a result of the systemic inflammatory response following surgery. The microglial cells up regulate the production of pro-inflammatory cytokines, which lead to disturbances in cognitive function and alterations in cerebral activity. In addition, over-activation of microglial cells can lead to neuronal apoptosis [10]. Thus, understanding the cellular and molecular pathways associated with microglial physiology may provide opportunities for intervention and targeted therapy for delirium treatment.

Endothelial cells serve as integral components of a competent blood brain barrier; however, in the setting of stress, surgery, inflammation, etc., endothelial function is altered leading to a reduction in the integrity of the highly selective blood brain barrier. This increases the risk of cerebral dysfunction and delirium development. Hughes et al. assessed biomarkers associated with the integrity of the blood brain barrier and endothelial dysfunction, and found that elevations in S1008, E-selectin and plasminogen activator-1 were associated with delirium in critical illness [12]. Endothelial dysfunction also up-regulates the coagulation pathways leading to microvascular thrombi formation, which consequently alters cerebral blood flow further leading to cerebral dysfunction.

Delirium is also linked to neurotransmitter dysfunction and deregulation. Acetylcholine is an important modulator of the systemic inflammatory response by decreasing the number of inflammatory cytokines. Critical illness and surgical stress create a physiologic environment that leads to depletion of acetylcholine stores and availability. A lack of acetylcholine receptor activation on the surface of microglial cells causes a lack of inhibition and leads to hyperactivation of microglial cells [10]. The acetylcholine association with delirium explains the pathophysiology involved with the increased risk of delirium in patients receiving anti-cholinergic medications. These medications exacerbate the depleted stores of acetylcholine that is associated with stress and post-surgical states. Hence, an important component of post-operative delirium prevention is to avoid the use of anti-cholinergic medications.

Additional neurotransmitter imbalances associated with the development of delirium include dopamine, serotonin, and norepinephrine [1, 10]. Elevated levels of dopamine and norepinephrine are associated with hyperactive delirium [13]. Increased norepinephrine levels contribute to agitation, impaired attention and cerebral dysfunction. Increased serotonin levels are also linked to cerebral dysfunction and increased risk of delirium. Gamma-aminobutyric acid (GABA) is the primary neurotransmitter associated with inhibitory pathways in the brain. Dysregulation of GABA is associated with delirium. The administration of drugs that are mechanistically involved in activation or inhibition of the GABA receptor or altering levels of other important neurotransmitters are associated with delirium, and efforts should be made to minimize patient exposure to these medications, such as benzodiazepines [13].

Overall, the pathophysiology linked to delirium is complex and incompletely understood. Importantly, delirium is the clinical manifestation that results from the interaction of multiple different dysfunctional systemic and cerebral physiologic pathways. As the understanding of the pathophysiology that leads to delirium improves, targeted pharmacologic agents can be developed and tested in clinical scenarios.

2. Diagnosis

2.1 Risk factors

Delirium is a very common complication following transplantation. It is important to have an appreciation for the risk factors linked to delirium development in order to optimize preventive measures and allow for early diagnosis. Advancing age and baseline cognitive impairment are the most commonly described risk factors for developing delirium [14, 15]. Certain medical conditions can also predispose patients to delirium. Sleep apnea, heart failure, diabetes and frailty have been shown to increase the risk of developing delirium [16]. Patients with lower cognitive and functional reserve likely have a reduced ability to maintain normal brain function in the setting of an acute stress event, such as surgery, sepsis or trauma. It is important to identify these risk factors that are present pre-operatively to help reduce the prevalence of delirium after transplant.

If cognitive dysfunction can predispose patients to delirium, an important question to answer when discussing delirium in transplant recipients is if surgery and/or anesthesia is an independent risk factor for post-operative cognitive defects (i.e. an unmodifiable risk factor for transplant recipients). A multicenter, prospective cohort study involving patients with surgical and nonsurgical critical illness was performed to evaluate if surgery and anesthesia was a risk factor for delirium. This study reported that surgery/anesthesia was not a risk factor for impairment of long-term global cognitive function or executive function after major non-cardiac surgery. In addition, increasing the level of exposure as measured by number of surgeries and duration of anesthesia was not associated with worse global cognitive or executive function. Cognitive impairment was highly prevalent at 3 and 12 months after hospital discharge in patients who suffered delirium. However, delirious patients who were exposed to general anesthesia and surgery suffered cognitive impairment at rates similar to those who did not undergo a surgical procedure. Post-operative cognitive impairment was associated with pre-existing cognitive deficits and level of education [3]. Based on these data, surgery and anesthesia does not appear to be an independent risk factor for delirium development and emphasizes the need for patient- and disease-focused risk stratification as transplant patients have many disease-specific risk factors that increase the incidence of delirium.

Risk factors for delirium in patients undergoing liver transplantation include a history of alcohol abuse, pre-operative hepatic encephalopathy, pre-operative renal replacement therapy, intra-operative red blood cell transfusion volume and increasing Acute Physiologic and Chronic Health Evaluation II (APACHE II) scores upon intensive care unit admission. A study by Wang et al. showed that risk factors associated with delirium in liver transplant patients in the intensive care unit included history of alcohol abuse (Odds ratio: 6.40), preoperative hepatic encephalopathy (Odds ratio: 4.45), APACHE II score > 16 (Odds ratio: 1.73), and duration of endotracheal intubation for >5 days (Odds ratio: 1.81) [17]. Lescot et al. performed an observational study of liver transplant patients admitted to the intensive care unit after deceased donor transplant. Neither age nor etiology of cirrhosis was significantly associated with delirium [18]. Furthermore, delirium was not significantly associated with Model for End Stage Liver Disease score or Child-Pugh score. The median number of intraoperative transfused packed red blood cell units in patients with delirium was more than double that of in patients without delirium ($P = 0.001$). The risk of developing delirium was greater in patients with pre-transplant encephalopathy ($P = 0.02$) and in patients who underwent renal replacement therapy during the pretransplantation period ($P < 0.01$). In the logistic regression model, number of red blood cell transfusions, renal replacement therapy, and elevated APACHE scores were associated with increased risk of delirium. Interestingly, if a patient required renal replacement therapy, they had 13-fold greater odds of becoming delirious [18].

Haugen et al. evaluated 893 kidney transplant recipients and examined risk factors for developing postoperative delirium [9]. Risk factors in patients with end stage renal disease undergoing kidney transplantation include age greater than 65 (Odds ratio: 2.65, $P = 0.004$), frail patients (Odds ratio: 2.05, $P = 0.04$), and increasing comorbidities (two or more on the Charlson Comorbidity Index) (Odds ratio: 1.93 $P = 0.05$). In regards to delirium in pancreas transplant recipients, there are currently no organ specific factors detailed in the literature; however, the known risk factors for delirium associated with patients undergoing kidney transplantation can be theoretically applied to pancreas transplant recipients as these patients share similar demographics and disease processes.

Post-operative factors that contribute to delirium include inadequate pain control, need for mechanical ventilation, sedation levels, benzodiazepine use, poor sleep hygiene, electrolyte disturbances, and infections. Medication used to treat common post-operative symptoms such as nausea including prochlorperazine or phenergan are associated with delirium. Benzodiazepines are also strongly associated with a higher risk of delirium and should only be used in very select circumstances at reduced doses in young patients with chronic home benzodiazepine use. Opioids increase delirium risk and should be used in moderation. Pain control should focus on multimodal treatment protocols with opioid sparing when applicable. Medications that alter the cholinergic neurotransmitter pathway, such as diphenhydramine, promethazine, tricyclic antidepressants or prochlorperazine are strongly associated with delirium development and should be avoided. In addition, immunosuppressive medications, such as calcineurin inhibitors and steroids, can be associated with mental status changes [19]. In transplant recipients at high risk for developing delirium or patients who have developed delirium, an important step in managing and optimizing these patients is to review the medication list to limit and discontinue any deliriogenic medication.

2.2 Screening

Early diagnosis of post-operative delirium is paramount for prompt management and minimization of risk for improved speed of recovery. There are several validated screening tools for assessing for the presence of delirium. The gold standard for diagnosis of delirium is a formal evaluation performed by a psychiatrist using The Diagnostic and Statistical Manual of Mental Disorders criteria; however, the application and feasibility of a formal psychiatric evaluation is not clinically practical [1]. More commonly used methods of delirium screening utilize nursing expertise for frequent and consistent bedside screening. The Richmond Agitation Sedation Scale (RASS) is a widely used screening tool to evaluate and communicate patients' level of sedation and arousal [20]. With an appropriate level of consciousness, there are many validated tools for delirium screening. Importantly, a patient must be arousable to voice (i.e. RASS score of −1) to be able to screen for delirium. The most commonly used tool for screening is the Confusion Assessment Method for Intensive Care Unit (CAM-ICU) [21]. The CAM-ICU (**Figure 2**) is an abbreviated version of the Confusion Assessment Method. The CAM-ICU tool screens for acute changes in mental status, inattention, disorganized thinking and altered level of consciousness in a condensed approach ideal for a fast paced clinical setting. The CAM-intensive care unit screening tool requires less than 2 min to complete and in addition to being rapidly applied, has been shown to be 93% sensitive and 98% specific for diagnosing delirium [21].

Other screening tools include the Nursing Delirium Symptom Checklist (NuDESC) [22], Confusion Assessment method (CAM) [23] and the Intensive Care Delirium Screening Checklist (ICDSC) [24]. The multiple, validated tools available speaks to the importance for using a tool of any type to achieve consistent screening. More important than which tool to use is having a program in place for regular, routine, and consistent screening. If delirium is not screened for using a validated screening tool, delirium may be missed up to 75% of the time [25–28], especially in the setting of hypoactive delirium. Given the fluctuating course of critically

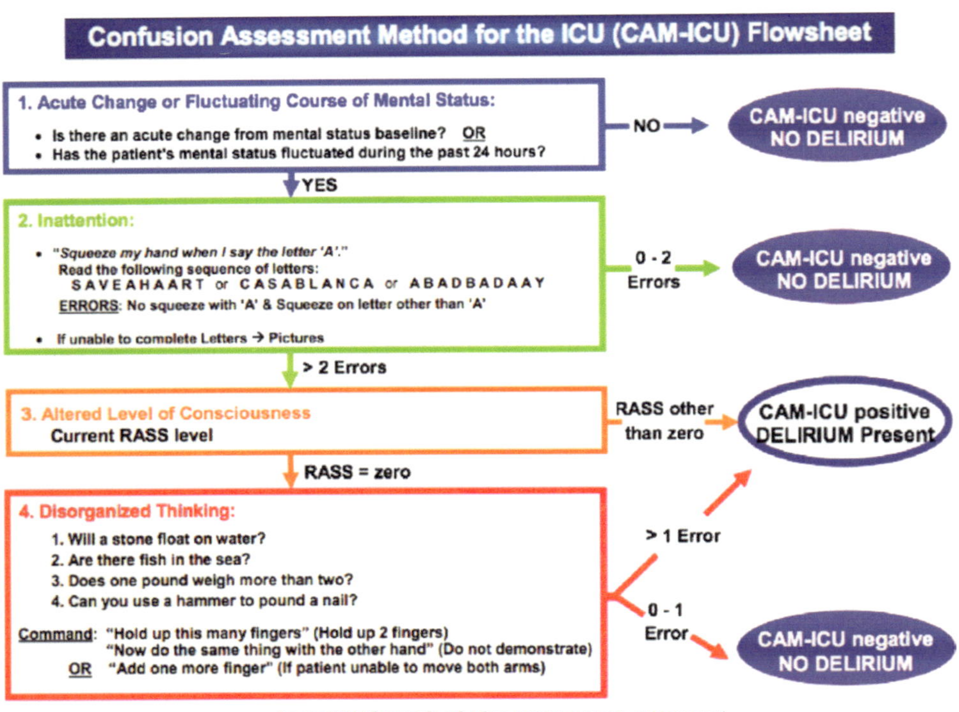

Figure 2.
Delirium screening tool and flowchart outlining the confusion assessment method for the intensive care unit [2].

ill patients and delirium, it is important that screening be performed in a serial, repeatable and consistent manner to achieve timely diagnosis and prevent under diagnosis. Routine implementation of validated screening tools allows for rapid and dependable evaluation and subsequent work up to identify potential underlying etiologies and ultimately directed delirium management.

2.3 Delirium work up

Following a positive screening evaluation for delirium, working through a differential diagnosis to identify treatable underlying causes is essential. In the transplant population in the setting of immunosuppression, infection is an extremely important diagnosis to consider and rule out in a timely manner. Immunosuppressed patients do not have a robust systemic inflammatory response as compared to non-immunosuppressed, post-operative patients, so infections present in a more discreet and subtle manner, often with mental status changes as the only clinical symptomatology. In a patient with new onset delirium, initial work up should include a comprehensive laboratory evaluation including a complete blood count, comprehensive metabolic panel, liver function tests, lipase and amylase. In the post-transplant recipient where renal dysfunction and electrolyte fluctuations are common, a basic metabolic panel should also be obtained to ensure that uremia or an underlying electrolyte disturbance is not present. Hormone dysregulation should also be considered as a cause of delirium with laboratory evaluation of thyroid function and the pituitary–adrenal axis. The patient's medication list should also be reviewed to ensure that medication toxicity is not contributing or exacerbating the mental status changes. However, in the immunosuppressed, post-operative transplant recipient with clinical decompensation highlighted by new onset mental status changes, sepsis needs to be at the top of the differential diagnosis.

Mental status changes are often the initial presenting symptom of an underlying infection or sepsis in the transplant population. Blood cultures, urine cultures, and a chest x-ray should be obtained to rule out bacteremia, urinary tract infection or pneumonia, respectively. In addition, based on the operative details and time since surgery, cross sectional axial imaging should be considered to rule out a deep space infection or other possible surgical complications. Importantly, early initiation of broad-spectrum antibiotics is strongly recommended if there is any concern that an underlying infection is contributing to the mental status changes.

If surgical drains are present, evaluating the character of the abdominal fluid is important to rule out intra-abdominal pathology. Organ specific evaluation of surgical drains is an important step in evaluating for potential infectious sources. In the setting of liver transplant, drains should be evaluated for elevated bilirubin to rule out a biloma and anastomotic biliary complication. In pancreas recipients, drain amylase and bilirubin should be obtained to evaluate for a pancreatic parenchyma leak and/or an enteric anastomotic leak. If clinically applicable in kidney transplant recipients, drain fluid should be checked for creatinine to evaluate for a possible urine leak. Drain fluid studies should be correlated with high resolution, axial imaging to further define the anatomic location of potential fluid collections to determine if percutaneous drainage or open drainage is needed.

Furthermore, the work up should include placing the patient on a pulse oximeter to obtain an oxygen saturation and obtain an arterial blood gas to ensure that hypoxia or hypercarbia is not causing or contributing to the mental status changes.

Myocardial infarctions and cerebral vascular events can also present with delirium. An electrocardiography, troponins and a possible echocardiography should be obtained if there is a concern for a cardiac event. If there is clinical suspicion for a stroke based on neurologic exam, a non-contrast and subsequently contrasted cerebral, cross sectional imaging should be obtained. In addition, an electroencephalography should be performed if there is clinical concern for seizure activity or postictal metal status changes.

Mental status changes in the transplant recipient can be caused by multiple contributing factors, and a systematic and thoughtful work up is paramount for rapid initiation of treatment. However, the work up for delirium is often negative for any treatable, underlying medical condition. Once all potential medical conditions that can contribute to delirium are evaluated and eliminated as the diagnosis, the focus should shift to optimizing the environment for delirium resolution and cognitive recovery.

3. Prevention

3.1 Pre-operative prevention

Surgery can result in accelerated cognitive and functional decline, and this cognitive impairment after surgery has been associated with increased mortality and disability with deficits in activities of daily living occurring in up to 50% of patients even 12 months after major surgery [29–34]. Patients with a higher physical and cognitive reserve have a protective effect on reducing the risk of developing delirium [35, 36]. Therapeutic approaches for improving cognitive reserve may present opportunities for reducing cognitive impairment after acute stressors, particularly in situations with time available for prehabilitation. An area that is understudied in the transplant population is whether building patients' mental and physical reserve through a prescribed program of cognitive and physical exercise, as well as nutritional optimization can improve long term outcomes. Prehabilitation efforts before surgery thus far have focused on preemptive physical therapy to improve post-surgical functional outcomes. Multiple studies have demonstrated that physical training prior to surgery to build physical reserve can improve functional outcomes after major surgery [37–39]. No work, however, has been done to attenuate the cognitive decline by "exercising the brain" before the physiologic insult that is commonly seen in chronic disease and surgical intervention such as transplantation.

By targeting high-risk individuals, such as those who are frail, encephalopathic, uremic, have a history of alcohol abuse, are of advanced age, and have higher Model for End Stage Liver Disease scores, cognitive reserve could be improved. There are interventions focused on cognitive remediation/rehabilitation that are being studied, which potentially hold promise for improving long-term brain functioning in transplant recipients. Among them, Cognitive Retraining is a novel therapeutic approach. Conceptually, Cognitive Retraining applies well-understood techniques derived from brain plasticity research [40]. The learning theory facilitates improvement in information processing, attention control, aspects of memory, and executive functioning. Research has been performed evaluating the effectiveness of computer-based cognitive remediation on various aspects of neuropsychological functioning including memory, attention, processing speed, and others [41–43]. Based on prior experience with a wide variety of patient populations, there is a high likelihood of fostering improvement in patient outcomes in transplant recipients if applied to high risk individuals at risk for cognitive impairment and delirium during their postoperative recovery.

3.2 Intra-operative management

It is extremely important for anesthesia providers to practice delirium preventive strategies. There are operative factors that need to be considered that are associated with increased delirium, which include the use of anticholinergic medications, electrolyte disturbances (specifically sodium fluctuations), and the amount of red blood cell transfusions. Efforts to decrease the prevalence of postoperative delirium should focus on limiting patient exposure to deliriogenic medications intra-operatively. The choice of anesthetic does not increase the risk of delirium as there is no conclusive evidence that propofol versus an inhaled based anesthetic changes the incidence of post-operative delirium [44, 45]. However, the level/depth of sedation provided during the operation is associated with delirium development, and therefore instruments such as intra-operative electroencephalography or brain activity monitors have been suggested to mitigate excessive levels of anesthesia helping with delirium prevention post-operatively. [46]. Close attention to electrolyte concentrations and fluctuations intraoperatively is also important. This is especially critical in patients with chronic hyponatremia, and in operations that involve large volume crystalloid resuscitation or excessive blood loss with associated blood product administration. Detailed pre-operative planning to minimize large fluctuations and optimize electrolyte disturbances should be performed with the surgical and anesthesia teams in high-risk individuals. Intra-operative management is an important part of the continuum of care for the transplant patient in delirium prevention.

3.3 Post-operative prevention

3.3.1 Pharmacologic prophylaxis

Studies evaluating whether pharmacologic prophylaxis reduced the incidence of delirium have shown mixed results. A large double blind, placebo controlled trial studied prophylactic dexmedetomidine infusion upon arrival to the intensive care unit. The intervention group demonstrated a significant reduction in the incidence of delirium in non-cardiac post-operative elderly patients compared to the control group [47]. Treatment with dexmedetomidine in elderly patients admitted to the intensive care unit after non-cardiac surgery reduced the incidence of delirium from 23 to 9%. Dexmedetomidine also reduced the amount of sedative drugs including narcotics administered. The authors suggested that the delirium reduction seen in the trial could be contributed to a possible neuroprotective effect of dexmedetomidine and/or a reduction in sedation medications. Wide spread clinical use of dexmedetomidine is limited by the fact that it must be used in in an intensive care setting being administered intravenously, as well as the possible cardiopulmonary side effect profile causing respiratory depression, hypotension and bradycardia. However, these results are encouraging for the use of dexmedetomidine in the prophylactic setting in patients at high risk for delirium.

There are no data on the use dexmedetomidine use in patients admitted to the intensive care unit following abdominal transplant, but this approach could be applicable to liver transplant patients who remain intubated at the time of intensive care unit admission to be used as sedation instead of fentanyl or propofol. Further work will need to be done to delineate a clinical benefit for routine use of dexmedetomidine in postoperative transplant patients.

A recent randomized controlled trial-The Haloperidol Effectiveness in ICU Delirium (HOPE-ICU) study-showed no difference in days alive and free of delirium between patients prophylactically treated with intravenous haloperidol (2.5 mg every 8 hours) or placebo [48]. At this time, the data are not conclusive to make a formal recommendation for routine pharmacologic prophylaxis for delirium prevention.

3.3.2 Non-pharmacologic prevention

Implementing non-pharmacologic based prevention bundles for delirium reduction have resulted in improved rates of delirium. The clinical care bundles focus on reducing exposure to and mitigating delirium risk factors such as appropriate pain management, timely Foley catheter removal, re-orientation strategies, and reducing hearing and vision deficits. Implementation of these protocols has reduced delirium rates and total days of delirium in multiple studies [49–51]. There is a growing emphasis on a multimodal approach to pain control to reduce exposure to deliriogenic narcotic pain medication. Multimodal pain control emphasizes opioid reduction with the use of a combination of acetaminophen, non-steroidal anti-inflammatory medications, ketamine, gabapentin and/or regional anesthetic techniques where appropriate. A multi-disciplinary approach with anesthesia, pain specialists and the surgical team should be implemented to optimize post-operative pain control with narcotic avoidance/reduction protocols.

Combining evidence-based interventions that reduce delirium rates have been shown to be effective and the combination of different strategies can have additive beneficial effects on delirium prevention. The Awakening and Breathing Coordination, Delirium Monitoring/Management, and Early Mobility (ABCDE) bundle is the most described bundle in the literature (**Figure 3**). Initially published in 2011 [52], this bundle has proven to be an effective strategy in delirium prevention. The ABCDE bundle is comprised of a number of interventions shown to improve outcomes in several well-designed clinical trials. The ABCDE bundle is an evidence-based, multicomponent management strategy aimed at reducing sedation exposure, duration of mechanical ventilation and hospital-acquired delirium and weakness. In comparison to standard practice including spontaneous breathing trials and spontaneous awakening trials (but no consistent delirium screening), the ABCDE bundle group experienced less delirium (48.7 vs. 62.3%, $P = 0.02$) and a lower percent of intensive care unit days spent delirious (33 vs. 50%, $P = 0.002$) [53]. The "AB" component of the bundle focuses on expedited mechanical ventilation liberation, and has been shown to decrease duration of medical ventilation, duration of coma and mortality [54, 55]. The "C" of the bundle is focused on avoiding over sedation and use of benzodiazepines, which has been shown in clinical trials to decrease delirium and duration of mechanical ventilation [56–58]. The "D" of the bundle refers to regular delirium screening and monitoring. The "E" of the bundle highlights the need for early mobility, which has been shown to decrease duration of delirium, intensive care unit length of stay and mortality [59]. A recent prospective, cohort study evaluated the effects of the ABCDE bundle on delirium rates. After the bundle was implemented, the prevalence of delirium decreased significantly from 38 to 23% ($P = 0.01$). The number of days with delirium was also reduced from 3.8 to 1.72 days ($P = <0.001$) [60]. These data support a focused, clinical care bundle approach to delirium prevention and prospective implementation in postoperative solid organ transplant recipients.

4. Treatment and management

4.1 Management

Most of the data exploring practice recommendations for delirium management is rooted in the critical care literature. Over the past two decades, significant shifts in practice paradigms have helped reduce the incidence of delirium in the intensive care unit. The major advancements in delirium management and prevention include

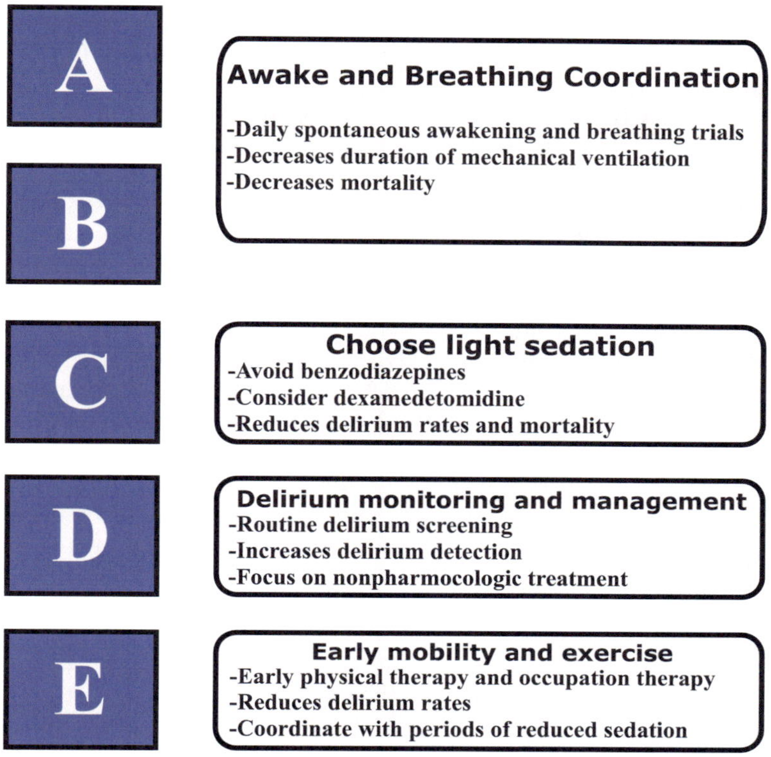

Figure 3.
Overview of the ABCDE delirium prevention bundle.

the level of sedation delivered while receiving mechanical ventilation. Daily awakening trials where sedation is interrupted to evaluate the ability to liberate from mechanical ventilation coupled with spontaneous breathing trials has been shown in randomized controlled studies to reduce mechanical ventilation days as well as delirium incidence [54, 61].

In addition, the choice of medication for sedation has shifted from benzodiazepines to propofol or dexmedetomidine infusions. This management shift was based on randomized controlled studies evaluating delirium outcomes and rates in patients receiving dexmedetomidine versus lorazepam infusions for sedation. Longer duration of lorazepam exposure was significantly associated with increased rates of delirium [57]. This study of 106 critically ill patients found that the patients receiving dexmedetomidine had more delirium free days compared to the lorazepam group (7 vs. 3, P = 0.01). Not only does duration of benzodiazepine exposure increase the incidence of delirium, it has been shown that delirium risk increases with amount of lorazepam administered [62].

An unintended consequence of routine intensive care unit care is sleep disruption and interference with sleep quality. Fragmented sleep has been associated with delirium. A focus on promoting and maintaining adequate sleep hygiene is an important delirium preventive measure. Efforts to minimize overnight disruptions and promote normal circadian rhythms have been associated with lower odds of developing delirium. Non-pharmacologic measures should be implemented to aid in sleep quality improvement and maintenance of sleep hygiene such as exposure to natural light, activity/mobility during the day, reduction of nighttime noise, removal of nocturnal stimulation, and reductions in night time nursing disruptions. A quality improvement project aimed at improving sleep by minimizing sleep disruptions and promoting normal circadian rhythms using non-pharmacological sleep aids has been shown to decrease the incidence of delirium and improve daily delirium free status [63].

Early mobilization is also an important strategy for delirium prevention. A trial of early mobilization that randomized hemodynamically stable patients to daily sedation interruptions timed with physical and occupation therapy versus usual care without early mobilization therapy achieved a two-day reduction in delirium duration in the treatment arm (days with delirium: 2 vs. 4 days, P = 0.03) [59]. In addition, early mobilization in this study reduced the time in the intensive care unit with delirium (33% of patients in the intervention group were diagnosed with delirium vs. 57% of patients in the control group were diagnosed with delirium, P = 0.02), as well as time in the hospital with delirium (28% of patients in the intervention group were diagnosed with delirium vs. 41% of patients in the control group were diagnosed with delirium, P = 0.01). Therapy included passive range of motion, active range of motion, and activities of daily living training depending on the patients' level of sedation and ability. In another recent randomized controlled trial of surgical critically ill patients, early goal-directed mobilization reduced the incidence of delirium and increased the number of delirium free days in the intensive care unit when compared to usual care [64].

4.2 Pharmacologic treatment

Currently, there are no evidence-based guidelines regarding specific pharmacological agents for delirium treatment. The current first line agents used in the treatment of hyperactive delirium are antipsychotic medications including haloperidol, olanzapine and quetiapine. Of note, neither antipsychotics nor dexmedetomidine have FDA approval for the treatment of delirium. In an international survey of 1521 intensivists, 65% reported that they treat delirium in the intensive care unit with haloperidol and 53% reported that they treat delirium with atypical antipsychotic medications [65], but there is no evidence-based literature showing efficacy of these medications for delirium treatment and symptom resolution. Despite current practice patterns, there are few data to support their definitive use in treating delirium.

A recent study evaluating the treatment of delirium with haloperidol (2.5–5 mg every 8 h) versus olanzapine (5 mg daily) showed no difference in length of delirium in 73 critically ill patients [66]. Furthermore, in a randomized, double blind, placebo-controlled trial, patients with acute respiratory failure or shock and hypoactive or hyperactive delirium were assigned to receive intravenous boluses of haloperidol (maximum dose, 20 mg daily), ziprasidone (maximum dose, 40 mg daily), or placebo [67]. The primary end point was the number of days alive without delirium or coma during the 14-day intervention period. The use of haloperidol or ziprasidone, as compared with placebo, in patients with acute respiratory failure or shock and hypoactive or hyperactive delirium in the intensive care unit did not significantly alter the duration of delirium. This randomized, placebo-controlled trial of intravenous antipsychotic medications for the treatment of delirium in critically ill patients showed that pharmacologic treatment was no different than placebo [67].

Dexmedetomidine in delirium management has gained popularity over the past several years. A recent trial studied dexmedetomidine in mechanically ventilated patients who were unable to be weaned from mechanical ventilation due to hyperactive delirium. This study, Dexmedetomidine to Lessen ICU Agitation trial, randomized patients to receive 7 days of intravenous dexmedetomidine (up to 1.5 μg/kg/h) or placebo. Patients treated with dexmedetomidine had fewer days requiring ventilator support and had faster resolution of delirium symptoms (23 vs. 40 h, P = 0.01) [68]. Dexmedetomidine must be administered as an infusion, which means the drug can only be given to patients having critical care needs. Alternative oral alpha-2 agonists exist, including clonidine or guanfacine, which could facilitate therapy in non- intensive care unit settings or during transition of care. However, these agents have not been rigorously studied in regards to delirium treatment and prevention as options for oral transition or alternatives to dexmedetomidine.

As strong evidence supporting the use of single pharmacological agents in delirium is lacking, preventive strategies and non-pharmacologic treatment bundles, such as the ABCDE bundle as discussed above, should be incorporated into delirium prevention and management algorithms.

4.3 Cognitive therapy following delirium

Cognitive and physical dysfunction is a common sequela for patients following a prolonged course of delirium. Recently, efforts have been made to minimize the long-term effects of delirium through exercises focused on orientation, memory, attention, and problem solving. A recent study implemented a graded cognitive therapy protocol with varying degrees of intensity guided by the patient's RASS assessment immediately preceding the session [69]. Examples of the cognitive therapy performed in this study included matrix puzzles, noun list recall, paragraph recall, letter-number sequence, and pattern recognition. The authors showed that following discharge from the intensive care unit, combined cognitive and physical therapy was associated with improved executive functioning at the time of hospital discharge [69]. These data suggest that once a patient is able to participate in therapy following delirium recovery, efforts should be made to incorporate cognitive rehabilitation as an integral part of the recovery process to maximize functional outcomes.

Extending beyond inpatient rehabilitation, research has been conducted into performing cognitive rehabilitation following hospital discharge in patients who suffered from delirium [70]. In this study the rehabilitation program was provided over a 12-week period after discharge in each patient's home and integrated both traditional "face-to-face" interventions as well as telephone and video-based interventions for cognitive, physical and functional rehabilitation. The cognitive training was based on the goal-management training (GMT) protocol, a focused and theoretically derived stepwise approach to the rehabilitation of executive function. The GMT sessions build on one another to increase the "dose" of rehabilitation delivered. These cognitive sessions resulted in improved scoring on tests evaluating executive functioning [70].

Based on studies in non-transplant populations, it would appear that transplant patients could similarly benefit from both inpatient and outpatient cognitive rehabilitation following delirium recovery in order to optimize long-term outcomes and maximize quality of life following transplantation.

As patients are recovering from delirium and transitioning to cognitive rehabilitation, it is important to focus on the completion of the treatment for any underlying condition, like sepsis, that lead to or contributed to delirium development to ensure optimal functional recovery.

5. Outcomes

Delirium in the postoperative setting significantly impacts outcomes. Delirium is a predictor of mortality in hospitalized patients [61], and mortality increases with the duration of delirium [71]. The relative hazard of death is nearly four times greater if a patient has delirium for 3 days versus no delirium. Beyond mortality, delirium also impacts quality of life following recovery. Delirium has been shown to negatively impact long-term cognitive function [72]. A recent multicenter, prospective, cohort study of critically ill patients was evaluated to estimate the prevalence of long-term cognitive impairment after critical illness [2]. The study enrolled adults with respiratory failure or shock in the medical or surgical intensive care unit, evaluated them for in-hospital delirium, and assessed global cognitive and executive function 3 and 12 months after discharge with the use of the Repeatable Battery for the Assessment of Neuropsychological Status. The study showed that one out of four patients had cognitive impairment 12 months after critical illness that was similar in severity to that of patients with mild Alzheimer's disease. At 3 months, 40% of the patients had global cognition scores that were 1.5 standard deviations below the population means (similar to scores for patients with moderate traumatic brain injury), and 26% had scores 2 standard deviations below the population means (similar to scores for patients with mild Alzheimer's disease). Interestingly, the degree of cognitive impairment affected older and younger patients equally. A longer duration of delirium was independently associated with worse global cognition at 3 and 12 months ($P = 0.001$ and $P = 0.04$, respectively) and worse executive function at 3 and 12 months [2]. These data strongly support efforts to initiate cognitive rehabilitation programs for patients who suffer from delirium during the postoperative period to enhance functional outcomes.

In regards to transplant specific outcomes in patients who suffer from delirium, Lescot et al. examined postoperative outcomes for patients with and without delirium following liver transplant [18]. Patients who suffered from delirium after liver transplant had higher rates of sepsis during the intensive care unit stay (18 vs. 1.2%, $P \leq 0.001$), longer days requiring mechanical ventilation (2 vs. 1, $P \leq 0.001$), longer intensive care unit length of stay (9 vs. 4 days, $P \leq 0.001$), and longer hospital length of stay (37 vs. 20 days, $P \leq 0.001$). In addition, patients who developed delirium had increased mortality compared to those patients who did not suffer from delirium, both in the short-term as well as at 1 year following transplant (intensive care unit mortality: 10.7 vs. 2%, $P = 0.04$; in-hospital mortality: 25 vs. 6%; 1 year mortality: 32 vs. 12%, $P = 0.007$) [18]. A recent prospective cohort study to evaluate postoperative delirium after liver transplantation showed that 45% of recipients experience delirium with a median duration of 5 days [8]. Furthermore, postoperative delirium was associated with a four-fold increase in intensive care unit length of stay, a more than two-fold increase in hospital length of stay, and decreased survival probability at 1 year. The authors suggest that postoperative delirium should be considered a preventable clinical complication, and not just a predictive risk factor for worse outcomes in the liver transplant population [8]. Postoperative complications likely contribute to both increased rates of delirium and mortality, however, it is clear that delirium is associated with worse outcomes.

Haugen et al. recently evaluated 125,304 adult kidney transplant recipients between 1999 and 2015 as reported to the Organ Procurement and Transplantation Network and linked to Medicare claims by the US Renal Data System [9]. International Classification of Diseases 9 codes for delirium were identified from inpatient claims throughout the entire set of initial kidney transplant hospitalizations. Haugen and colleagues showed that delirium in kidney transplant recipients significantly associates with patient survival, with an approximately 40% mortality at 5 years for patients who developed delirium post transplant compared to 10% mortality for patients who did not suffer from delirium [9].

6. Summary

Delirium is a common clinical diagnosis in the solid organ transplant population. Delirium is under diagnosed, yet the recent appreciation of its impact on cognitive recovery indicates it is vital make efforts to mitigate its development and recognize it in a timely fashion to optimize transplant outcomes. Delirium has been shown to be associated with a longer length of stay, increased medical costs, increased morbidity/mortality and decreased cognitive function following hospital discharge. Non-pharmacologic preventive strategies, routine delirium screening, and performing a comprehensive evaluation for an underlying medical cause of delirium with prompt treatment are the cornerstones of delirium management. With a better understanding of the negative impact on both short and long term outcomes associated with delirium in the transplant population, a focused, multidisciplinary approach to delirium prevention and management strategies to decrease the prevalence and minimize duration of delirium is paramount in transplant recipients. Delirium should no longer be viewed as an unavoidable clinical complication in transplant patients. Instead, proactive measures for cognitive prehabilitation in high risk transplant candidates, together with the use of clinical prevention bundles and post-delirium rehabilitation programs are key components of maximizing patient survival and functional outcomes following solid organ transplantation.

Conflict of interest

The authors have no conflicts of interest to report.

Author details

Clark D. Kensinger* and Jon S. Odorico
Department of General Surgery, Division of Transplant, University of Wisconsin School of Medicine and Public Health, Madison, WI, USA

*Address all correspondence to: Kensinger@wisc.edu

References

[1] Rengel KF, Pandharipande PP, Hughes CG. Postoperative delirium. La Presse Médicale. 2018;**47**(4 Pt 2): e53-e64

[2] Pandharipande PP, Girard TD, Jackson JC, Morandi A, Thompson JL, Pun BT, et al. Long-term cognitive impairment after critical illness. The New England Journal of Medicine. 2013;**369**(14):1306-1316

[3] Hughes CG, Patel MB, Jackson JC, Girard TD, Geevarghese SK, Norman BC, et al. Surgery and anesthesia exposure is not a risk factor for cognitive impairment after major noncardiac surgery and critical illness. Annals of Surgery. 2017;**265**(6):1126-1133

[4] Robinson TN, Raeburn CD, Tran ZV, Brenner LA, Moss M. Motor subtypes of postoperative delirium in older adults. Archives of Surgery. 2011;**146**(3):295-300

[5] Vasilevskis EE, Han JH, Hughes CG, Ely EW. Epidemiology and risk factors for delirium across hospital settings. Best Practice and Research. Clinical Anaesthesiology. 2012;**26**(3):277-287

[6] Card E, Pandharipande P, Tomes C, Lee C, Wood J, Nelson D, et al. Emergence from general anaesthesia and evolution of delirium signs in the post-anaesthesia care unit. British Journal of Anaesthesia. 2015;**115**(3):411-417

[7] Bronster DJ, Emre S, Boccagni P, Sheiner PA, Schwartz ME, Miller CM. Central nervous system complications in liver transplant recipients—Incidence, timing, and long-term follow-up. Clinical Transplantation. 2000;**14**(1):1-7

[8] Beckmann S, Schubert M, Burkhalter H, Dutkowski P, De Geest S. Postoperative delirium after liver transplantation is associated with increased length of stay and lower survival in a prospective cohort. Progress in Transplantation (Aliso Viejo, California). 2017;**27**(1):23-30

[9] Haugen CE, Mountford A, Warsame F, Berkowitz R, Bae S, Thomas AG, et al. Incidence, risk factors, and sequelae of post-kidney transplant delirium. Journal of the American Society of Nephrology. 2018;**29**(6):1752-1759

[10] Hughes CG, Patel MB, Pandharipande PP. Pathophysiology of acute brain dysfunction: What's the cause of all this confusion? Current Opinion in Critical Care. 2012;**18**(5):518-526

[11] Gunther ML, Morandi A, Krauskopf E, Pandharipande P, Girard TD, Jackson JC, et al. The association between brain volumes, delirium duration, and cognitive outcomes in intensive care unit survivors: The VISIONS cohort magnetic resonance imaging study. Critical Care Medicine. 2012;**40**(7):2022-2032

[12] Hughes CG, Pandharipande PP, Thompson JL, Chandrasekhar R, Ware LB, Ely EW, et al. Endothelial activation and blood-brain barrier injury as risk factors for delirium in critically ill patients. Critical Care Medicine. 2016;**44**(9):e809-e817

[13] Maldonado JR. Neuropathogenesis of delirium: Review of current etiologic theories and common pathways. The American Journal of Geriatric Psychiatry. 2013;**21**(12):1190-1222

[14] Booka E, Kamijo T, Matsumoto T, Takeuchi M, Kitani T, Nagaoka M, et al. Incidence and risk factors for postoperative delirium after major head and neck cancer surgery. Journal of Cranio-Maxillo-Facial Surgery. 2016;**44**(7):890-894

[15] van der Sluis FJ, Buisman PL, Meerdink M, Aan de Stegge WB, van Etten B, de Bock GH, et al. Risk factors for postoperative delirium after colorectal operation. Surgery. 2017;**161**(3):704-711

[16] Brummel NE, Vasilevskis EE, Han JH, Boehm L, Pun BT, Ely EW. Implementing delirium screening in the ICU: Secrets to success. Critical Care Medicine. 2013;**41**(9):2196-2208

[17] Wang SH, Wang JY, Lin PY, Lin KH, Ko CJ, Hsieh CE, et al. Predisposing risk factors for delirium in living donor liver transplantation patients in intensive care units. PLoS One. 2014;**9**(5):e96676

[18] Lescot T, Karvellas CJ, Chaudhury P, Tchervenkov J, Paraskevas S, Barkun J, et al. Postoperative delirium in the intensive care unit predicts worse outcomes in liver transplant recipients. Canadian Journal of Gastroenterology. 2013;**27**(4):207-212

[19] Schreiber MP, Colantuoni E, Bienvenu OJ, Neufeld KJ, Chen KF, Shanholtz C, et al. Corticosteroids and transition to delirium in patients with acute lung injury. Critical Care Medicine. 2014;**42**(6):1480-1486

[20] Sessler CN, Gosnell MS, Grap MJ, Brophy GM, O'Neal PV, Keane KA, et al. The Richmond Agitation-Sedation scale: Validity and reliability in adult intensive care unit patients. The American Journal of Respiratory and Critical Care Medicine. 2002;**166**(10):1338-1344

[21] Ely EW, Inouye SK, Bernard GR, Gordon S, Francis J, May L, et al. Delirium in mechanically ventilated patients: Validity and reliability of the confusion assessment method for the intensive care unit (CAM-ICU). JAMA. 2001;**286**(21):2703-2710

[22] Gaudreau JD, Gagnon P, Harel F, Tremblay A, Roy MA. Fast, systematic, and continuous delirium assessment in hospitalized patients: The nursing delirium screening scale. Journal of Pain and Symptom Management. 2005;**29**(4):368-375

[23] Inouye SK, van Dyck CH, Alessi CA, Balkin S, Siegal AP, Horwitz RI. Clarifying confusion: The confusion assessment method. A new method for detection of delirium. Annals of Internal Medicine. 1990;**113**(12):941-948

[24] Bergeron N, Dubois MJ, Dumont M, Dial S, Skrobik Y. Intensive care delirium screening checklist: Evaluation of a new screening tool. Intensive Care Medicine. 2001;**27**(5):859-864

[25] Inouye SK, Foreman MD, Mion LC, Katz KH, Cooney LM Jr. Nurses' recognition of delirium and its symptoms: Comparison of nurse and researcher ratings. Archives of Internal Medicine. 2001;**161**(20):2467-2473

[26] Devlin JW, Fong JJ, Schumaker G, O'Connor H, Ruthazer R, Garpestad E. Use of a validated delirium assessment tool improves the ability of physicians to identify delirium in medical intensive care unit patients. Critical Care Medicine. 2007;**35**(12):2721-2724. quiz 2725

[27] Spronk PE, Riekerk B, Hofhuis J, Rommes JH. Occurrence of delirium is severely underestimated in the ICU during daily care. Intensive Care Medicine. 2009;**35**(7):1276-1280

[28] van Eijk MM, van Marum RJ, Klijn IA, de Wit N, Kesecioglu J, Slooter AJ. Comparison of delirium assessment tools in a mixed intensive care unit. Critical Care Medicine. 2009;**37**(6):1881-1885

[29] Steinmetz J, Christensen KB, Lund T, Lohse N, Rasmussen LS. Long-term consequences of postoperative cognitive dysfunction. Anesthesiology. 2009;**110**(3):548-555

[30] Newman MF, Kirchner JL, Phillips-Bute B, Gaver V, Grocott H, Jones RH, et al. Longitudinal assessment of neurocognitive function after coronary-artery bypass surgery. The New England Journal of Medicine. 2001;**344**(6):395-402

[31] Quinlan N, Rudolph JL. Postoperative delirium and functional decline after noncardiac surgery. Journal of the American Geriatrics Society. 2011;**59**(Suppl 2):S301-S304

[32] Saczynski JS, Marcantonio ER, Quach L, Fong TG, Gross A, Inouye SK, et al. Cognitive trajectories after postoperative delirium. The New England Journal of Medicine. 2012;**367**(1):30-39

[33] Liang CK, Chu CL, Chou MY, Lin YT, Lu T, Hsu CJ, et al. Interrelationship of postoperative delirium and cognitive impairment and their impact on the functional status in older patients undergoing orthopaedic surgery: A prospective cohort study. PLoS One. 2014;**9**(11):e110339

[34] Rudolph JL, Inouye SK, Jones RN, Yang FM, Fong TG, Levkoff SE, et al. Delirium: An independent predictor of functional decline after cardiac surgery. Journal of the American Geriatrics Society. 2010;**58**(4):643-649

[35] Jones RN, Fong TG, Metzger E, Tulebaev S, Yang FM, Alsop DC, et al. Aging, brain disease, and reserve: Implications for delirium. The American Journal of Geriatric Psychiatry. 2010;**18**(2):117-127

[36] Quinlan N, Marcantonio ER, Inouye SK, Gill TM, Kamholz B, Rudolph JL. Vulnerability: The crossroads of frailty and delirium. Journal of the American Geriatrics Society. 2011;**59**(Suppl 2): S262-S268

[37] Gillis C, Li C, Lee L, Awasthi R, Augustin B, Gamsa A, et al. Prehabilitation versus rehabilitation: A randomized control trial in patients undergoing colorectal resection for cancer. Anesthesiology. 2014;**121**(5):937-947

[38] Topp R, Swank AM, Quesada PM, Nyland J, Malkani A. The effect of prehabilitation exercise on strength and functioning after total knee arthroplasty. PM & R: The Journal of Injury, Function, and Rehabilitation. 2009;**1**(8):729-735

[39] Nielsen PR, Jorgensen LD, Dahl B, Pedersen T, Tonnesen H. Prehabilitation and early rehabilitation after spinal surgery: Randomized clinical trial. Clinical Rehabilitation. 2010;**24**(2):137-148

[40] Abbott A. Gaming improves multitasking skills. Nature. 2013;**501**(7465):18

[41] Smith GE, Housen P, Yaffe K, Ruff R, Kennison RF, Mahncke HW, et al. A cognitive training program based on principles of brain plasticity: Results from the improvement in memory with plasticity-based adaptive cognitive training (IMPACT) study. Journal of the American Geriatrics Society. 2009;**57**(4):594-603

[42] Edwards JD, Wadley VG, Vance DE, Wood K, Roenker DL, Ball KK. The impact of speed of processing training on cognitive and everyday performance. Aging and Mental Health. 2005;**9**(3):262-271

[43] Barnes DE, Yaffe K, Belfor N, Jagust WJ, DeCarli C, Reed BR, et al. Computer-based cognitive training for mild cognitive impairment: Results from a pilot randomized, controlled trial. Alzheimer Disease and Associated Disorders. 2009;**23**(3):205-210

[44] Royse CF, Andrews DT, Newman SN, Stygall J, Williams Z, Pang J, et al.

The influence of propofol or desflurane on postoperative cognitive dysfunction in patients undergoing coronary artery bypass surgery. Anaesthesia. 2011;**66**(6):455-464

[45] Tanaka P, Goodman S, Sommer BR, Maloney W, Huddleston J, Lemmens HJ. The effect of desflurane versus propofol anesthesia on postoperative delirium in elderly obese patients undergoing total knee replacement: A randomized, controlled, double-blinded clinical trial. Journal of Clinical Anesthesia. 2017;**39**:17-22

[46] Radtke FM, Franck M, Lendner J, Kruger S, Wernecke KD, Spies CD. Monitoring depth of anaesthesia in a randomized trial decreases the rate of postoperative delirium but not postoperative cognitive dysfunction. British Journal of Anaesthesia. 2013;**110**(Suppl 1):i98-i105

[47] Su X, Meng ZT, Wu XH, Cui F, Li HL, Wang DX, et al. Dexmedetomidine for prevention of delirium in elderly patients after non-cardiac surgery: A randomised, double-blind, placebo-controlled trial. Lancet. 2016;**388**(10054):1893-1902

[48] Page VJ, Ely EW, Gates S, Zhao XB, Alce T, Shintani A, et al. Effect of intravenous haloperidol on the duration of delirium and coma in critically ill patients (Hope-ICU): A randomised, double-blind, placebo-controlled trial. The Lancet Respiratory Medicine. 2013;**1**(7):515-523

[49] Siddiqi N, Harrison JK, Clegg A, Teale EA, Young J, Taylor J, et al. Interventions for preventing delirium in hospitalised non-ICU patients. The Cochrane Database of Systematic Reviews. 2016;**3**:Cd005563

[50] Inouye SK, Bogardus ST Jr, Charpentier PA, Leo-Summers L, Acampora D, Holford TR, et al. A multicomponent intervention to prevent delirium in hospitalized older patients. The New England Journal of Medicine. 1999;**340**(9):669-676

[51] Reston JT, Schoelles KM. In-facility delirium prevention programs as a patient safety strategy: A systematic review. Annals of Internal Medicine. 2013;**158**(5 Pt 2):375-380

[52] Morandi A, Brummel NE, Ely EW. Sedation, delirium and mechanical ventilation: The 'ABCDE' approach. Current Opinion in Critical Care. 2011;**17**(1):43-49

[53] Balas MC, Vasilevskis EE, Olsen KM, Schmid KK, Shostrom V, Cohen MZ, et al. Effectiveness and safety of the awakening and breathing coordination, delirium monitoring/management, and early exercise/mobility bundle. Critical Care Medicine. 2014;**42**(5):1024-1036

[54] Ely EW, Baker AM, Dunagan DP, Burke HL, Smith AC, Kelly PT, et al. Effect on the duration of mechanical ventilation of identifying patients capable of breathing spontaneously. The New England Journal of Medicine. 1996;**335**(25):1864-1869

[55] Kress JP, Pohlman AS, O'Connor MF, Hall JB. Daily interruption of sedative infusions in critically ill patients undergoing mechanical ventilation. The New England Journal of Medicine. 2000;**342**(20):1471-1477

[56] Strom T, Martinussen T, Toft P. A protocol of no sedation for critically ill patients receiving mechanical ventilation: A randomised trial. Lancet. 2010;**375**(9713):475-480

[57] Pandharipande PP, Pun BT, Herr DL, Maze M, Girard TD, Miller RR, et al. Effect of sedation with dexmedetomidine vs lorazepam on acute brain dysfunction in mechanically ventilated patients: The MENDS

randomized controlled trial. JAMA. 2007;**298**(22):2644-2653

[58] Riker RR, Shehabi Y, Bokesch PM, Ceraso D, Wisemandle W, Koura F, et al. Dexmedetomidine vs midazolam for sedation of critically ill patients: A randomized trial. JAMA. 2009;**301**(5):489-499

[59] Schweickert WD, Pohlman MC, Pohlman AS, Nigos C, Pawlik AJ, Esbrook CL, et al. Early physical and occupational therapy in mechanically ventilated, critically ill patients: A randomised controlled trial. Lancet. 2009;**373**(9678):1874-1882

[60] Bounds M, Kram S, Speroni KG, Brice K, Luschinski MA, Harte S, et al. Effect of ABCDE bundle implementation on prevalence of delirium in intensive care unit patients. The American Journal of Critical Care. 2016;**25**(6):535-544

[61] Ely EW, Shintani A, Truman B, Speroff T, Gordon SM, Harrell FE Jr, et al. Delirium as a predictor of mortality in mechanically ventilated patients in the intensive care unit. JAMA. 2004;**291**(14):1753-1762

[62] Pandharipande P, Shintani A, Peterson J, Pun BT, Wilkinson GR, Dittus RS, et al. Lorazepam is an independent risk factor for transitioning to delirium in intensive care unit patients. Anesthesiology. 2006;**104**(1):21-26

[63] Alexopoulou C, Kondili E, Diamantaki E, Psarologakis C, Kokkini S, Bolaki M, et al. Effects of dexmedetomidine on sleep quality in critically ill patients: A pilot study. Anesthesiology. 2014;**121**(4):801-807

[64] Schaller SJ, Anstey M, Blobner M, Edrich T, Grabitz SD, Gradwohl-Matis I, et al. Early, goal-directed mobilisation in the surgical intensive care unit: A randomised controlled trial. Lancet. 2016;**388**(10052):1377-1388

[65] Morandi A, Piva S, Ely EW, Myatra SN, Salluh JIF, Amare D, et al. Worldwide survey of the "Assessing pain, both spontaneous awakening and breathing trials, choice of drugs, delirium monitoring/ management, early exercise/ mobility, and family empowerment" (ABCDEF). Critical Care Medicine. 2017;**45**(11):e1111-e1122

[66] Skrobik YK, Bergeron N, Dumont M, Gottfried SB. Olanzapine vs haloperidol: Treating delirium in a critical care setting. Intensive Care Medicine. 2004;**30**(3):444-449

[67] Girard TD, Exline MC, Carson SS, Hough CL, Rock P, Gong MN, et al. Haloperidol and ziprasidone for treatment of delirium in critical illness. The New England Journal of Medicine. 2018;**379**(26):2506-2516

[68] Reade MC, Eastwood GM, Bellomo R, Bailey M, Bersten A, Cheung B, et al. Effect of dexmedetomidine added to standard care on ventilator-free time in patients with agitated delirium: A randomized clinical trial. JAMA. 2016;**315**(14):1460-1468

[69] Brummel NE, Girard TD, Ely EW, Pandharipande PP, Morandi A, Hughes CG, et al. Feasibility and safety of early combined cognitive and physical therapy for critically ill medical and surgical patients: The activity and cognitive therapy in ICU (ACT-ICU) trial. Intensive Care Medicine. 2014;**40**(3):370-379

[70] Jackson JC, Ely EW, Morey MC, Anderson VM, Denne LB, Clune J, et al. Cognitive and physical rehabilitation of intensive care unit survivors: Results of the RETURN randomized controlled pilot investigation. Critical Care Medicine. 2012;**40**(4):1088-1097

[71] Shehabi Y, Riker RR, Bokesch PM, Wisemandle W, Shintani A, Ely EW. Delirium duration and mortality in lightly sedated, mechanically ventilated intensive care patients. Critical Care Medicine. 2010;**38**(12):2311-2318

[72] Girard TD, Jackson JC, Pandharipande PP, Pun BT, Thompson JL, Shintani AK, et al. Delirium as a predictor of long-term cognitive impairment in survivors of critical illness. Critical Care Medicine. 2010;**38**(7):1513-1520